PODIATRIC ASSESSMENT AND MANAGEMENT OF THE DIABETIC FOOT

For Elsevier:

Commissioning Editor: Robert Edwards
Development: Veronika Krcilova
Project Manager: Joannah Duncan
Design: George Ajayi
Illustrations: Barking Dog

PODIATRIC ASSESSMENT AND MANAGEMENT OF THE DIABETIC FOOT

Alethea VM Foster BA(Hons) PGCE DPodM MChS

Honorary Consultant Podiatrist, King's College Hospital NHS Trust, London, UK

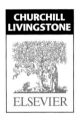

EDINBURGH LONDON NEW YORK OXFORD PHILADELPHIA
ST LOUIS SYDNEY TORONTO 2006

CHURCHILL
LIVINGSTONE
ELSEVIER

© 2006, Elsevier Limited. All rights reserved.
First published 2006

The right of Alethea Foster to be identified as author of this work has been asserted by her in accordance with the Copyright, Designs and Patents Act 1988.

ISBN 0 443 10043 8

British Library Cataloguing in Publication Data
A catalogue record for this book is available from the British Library.

Library of Congress Cataloging in Publication Data
A catalog record for this book is available from the Library of Congress.

Note
Knowledge and best practice in this field are constantly changing. As new research and experience broaden our knowledge, changes in practice, treatment and drug therapy may become necessary or appropriate. Readers are advised to check the most current information provided (i) on procedures featured or (ii) by the manufacturer of each product to be administered, to verify the recommended dose or formula, the method and duration of administration, and contraindications. It is the responsibility of the practitioner, relying on their own experience and knowledge of the patient, to make diagnoses, to determine dosages and the best treatment for each individual patient, and to take all appropriate safety precautions. To the fullest extent of the law, neither the Publisher nor the Author assumes any liability for any injury and/or damage to persons or property arising out of or related to any use of the material contained in this book.

The Publisher

Contents

This book is for Dr Michael Edmonds, consultant physician at the diabetic foot clinic, King's College Hospital. Mike is a great supporter of the podiatry profession and has been my mentor, my inspiration, and my generous guide.

Preface

Those wounds heal ill which men do give themselves.
Omission to do what is necessary,
Seals a commission to a blank of danger,
And danger, like an ague, subtly taints
Even then, when we sit idly in the sun …
William Shakespeare, Troilus and Cressida III. III. 230

This is a book for podiatrists and other healthcare professionals who have, or wish to develop, a particular interest in the diabetic foot. They may be students or they may already have many years of work experience and be only too aware of the enormous challenges faced by those who care for diabetic feet (Fig. 1).

In Europe, people with diabetes make up around 3% of the general population, yet half of all major amputations of a leg happen within this minority group, and similarly shocking statistics are to be found throughout the world. Diabetes is increasing in every country and in this still-new millennium we face an epidemic of diabetes. Along with this will come an epidemic of amputations, unless urgent steps are taken to improve diabetic foot care.

The aim of this book is to describe how podiatrists can achieve better outcomes for their diabetic patients, how amputations can be prevented with well-organized diabetic foot services, and how people with diabetes can be helped to avoid foot catastrophes. Not all diabetic foot problems can be prevented or healed, and sometimes major amputations are unavoidable, but in the majority of cases a better outcome can be achieved if patients gain early and sustained access to skilled, dedicated, and experienced podiatrists.

It is essential for podiatrists to understand how to examine, classify, and stage diabetic feet, and how to use their findings as a framework for choosing the most appropriate and effective treatments for their diabetic patients. They must know when to refer their patients on to other members of the healthcare team, and learn the best ways of working with, and gaining support from, other healthcare professionals in the field of diabetes, so that doctors,

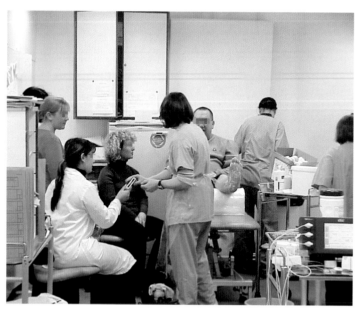

Fig. 1   In this busy scene from the multidisciplinary diabetic foot clinic at King's College Hospital, podiatrists and footcare assistants in surgical blues are working on the right, while student podiatrists from the University of Northampton and visiting podiatrists learn what it is like to assess and treat diabetic feet in the real world. The patient is awaiting a total contact cast for his acute Charcot foot and the student in a white coat is looking at the surface temperature of the foot, which has been recorded on an infrared thermometer. In the foreground is the transcutaneous oxymetry machine, used to ensure adequate perfusion of the foot that is about to be casted. The patient has previously been seen by the physician, the orthotist, and the orthopaedic surgeon. No one person can manage the high-risk diabetic foot: it takes a team.

nurses, surgeons, and orthotists also become supporters of podiatry and the diabetic foot.

The diabetic foot should never be treated as an island: to quote John Donne, it is 'a piece of the continent and a part of the main'. The podiatrist, equally, should not work in isolation but should be an integral part of the diabetes team.

It has often been said that no one person can handle every aspect of preventing and treating diabetic foot problems and that it takes a multidisciplinary team to reduce amputations. This is true, at least for the high-risk foot in diabetes, and one of the themes of this book is that it should be the podiatrist who stands at the heart of the team, manning the foot clinic, providing regular treatments, building relationships with patients and their families, acting as the first point of contact in an emergency situation, and knowing how, when, and where to obtain further help where necessary.

To succeed in their role within the diabetic foot team, podiatrists need to acquire extensive knowledge about diabetes to understand and support the work done by other members of the multidisciplinary diabetic foot team.

Problems can sometimes develop within groups. Just as there are many different roles for the podiatrist in diabetic foot care, so there is often overlap between the roles of the different members of the multidisciplinary diabetic foot team. Individual roles may depend on history, tradition, and the local situation, and this can sometimes lead to jealousy or disquiet if people feel that their own area of expertise is being invaded or usurped. Podiatrists may find it disconcerting when nurses want to learn sharp debridement techniques, and when podiatrists manufacture insoles and adjust footwear then orthotists may object. Some orthopaedic surgeons dislike working with or supporting podiatrists who have undergone postgraduate surgical training. It is essential not to allow interprofessional rivalries to erode relationships with other healthcare professionals within the team, as this will jeopardize good patient care.

It is my hope that this book will help podiatrists and other healthcare professionals to understand each other better, and to manage diabetic feet successfully wherever they encounter them. I also hope that by reading it, other members of the healthcare team will gain valuable insights into the role of the podiatrist.

My early days training and working as a podiatrist who always intended to specialize in diabetes, over 20 years ago, were frustrating in many respects. I remember my amazement at the lack of podiatry textbooks: we were taught at the patient's chair side, and from dictated notes. We only saw one or two neuropathic ulcers during our 3-year training; these were cautiously debrided by members of the teaching staff, who were very careful not to draw blood. I also well remember attending my first diabetic foot meeting, where a vascular surgeon put up a slide listing the causes of gangrene; chiropody was at the top of the list. Things have improved since then and in the twenty-first century, podiatry is better understood. However, podiatrists who intend to enter the field of diabetic foot management should be aware that the care of the high-risk diabetic foot is not a 'nine to five job' nor a bed of roses. Podiatrists wanting to specialize in this area need to be aware that the pathology is unrelenting and overwhelming. The acute diabetic foot in the United Kingdom has a curious propensity for presenting without warning at inconvenient times, including five o'clock on Friday afternoon and noon on Christmas Eve. This is not an area for the faint hearted. Enthusiasm, energy, and dedication are essential: podiatrists cannot afford to 'sit idly in the sun' while their patients' wounds fail to heal.

Fortunately, in addition to being demanding, the role of the specialist podiatrist in diabetes is also tremendously exciting and interesting. The high-risk diabetic foot is one of the greatest professional challenges that podiatrists will ever encounter. By managing it well, we can save lives and limbs, greatly improve the quality of life of our patients, and achieve great satisfaction in our work. However, the diabetic foot can be a deeply frustrating specialty if podiatrists fail to gain the confidence and support of colleagues in other healthcare specialties. Good interdisciplinary communications are essential and diabetic podiatrists should never work in isolation.

It is unfortunate that many British diabetic patients still find it impossible to obtain regular, sufficiently frequent podiatric treatment, or rapid help from an experienced diabetic foot team when problems develop. It is to be hoped that the new National Service Framework for Diabetes will help to improve diabetic foot services for people in the United Kingdom and that rapid access to podiatry and multidisciplinary diabetic foot clinics will gradually become available in all areas, and not remain, by 'postcode lottery', available only to a fortunate few.

Wherever possible, properly conducted research studies have been used as a basis for recommendations. However, there is a dearth of studies and many of the assertions in this book are therefore based on first-hand experience and additional information gleaned from respected colleagues over many years.

Throughout this book, the patient is referred to as 'he'. This is partly because the majority of diabetic foot patients are male but also because the author has a great aversion to 'political correctness'. For the same reason, patients are not called clients or customers, and terms such as 'counselling', 'proactive', 'judgemental', and others of that ilk have been avoided. The words 'non-compliant' are used to describe patients who, for whatever reason, do not follow advice. Podiatrists are referred to as 'she' because in the United Kingdom most podiatrists are women.

The International Diabetes Federation has designated 2005 as 'the year of the diabetic foot', and there is an ever-increasing demand for information and education in this exciting field. I hope that this very practical book will be useful for all members of the healthcare team who encounter diabetic feet during their working lives.

Alethea Foster
London 2006

Acknowledgements

During my twenty years at King's College Hospital, I have received a tremendous amount of help and encouragement from colleagues and patients, both in the hospital and the community, who are far too numerous to mention but who know who they are: thank you chaps.

During my work abroad I have always encountered great hospitality, warmth, and kindness from people all over the world, and Karel Bakker has been a great friend and supporter on the international scene: I am very grateful.

My podiatric colleagues at King's have encouraged and helped me with unstinting generosity and held the fort without complaining when I was away, so they deserve special mention. So, in chronological order, Cathy Eaton, Diane Birkinshaw, Mark Greenhill, Susie Spenser, Maureen Bates, Melanie Doxford, Lizzie Hampton, Tim Jemmott and Debbie Broome step forward and take a bow.

Writing books is hard on families so I also want to thank John, Jay, Will, Dennis, Rosemary, Pen, Alex, Lynda, Vicky, Bill, Cece, Brian, Bella, James, Suzanne, Henry, Christine and all my nephews and nieces for putting up with my neglect, without complaining, over the past few months.

Lastly, my gratitude goes to Robert Edwards at Elsevier, who commissioned this book, for his encouragement and support.

1 Why diabetic feet get into trouble

You knew he walked o'er perils, on an edge,
More likely to fall in than to get o'er;
You were advised his flesh was capable
Of wounds and scars, and that his forward spirit,
Would lift him where most trade of danger ranged.

William Shakespeare, Henry IV Part II. I. I. 170

The majority of patients begin their diabetic lives with 'normal' feet – although some patients with type 2 diabetes will have foot complications at diagnosis, that is only because they have been diabetic for many years without knowing it (because their symptoms were slight, or put down to the ageing process or other factors) (Fig. 1.1). However, normality covers a wide range of foot states and some conditions that would not give rise to serious problems in non-diabetic patients can cause grave trouble in diabetic feet. Moreover, even normal feet, if deprived of adequate foot care or incarcerated in unsuitable shoes, can develop long-term problems. Risk assessment and risk factor modification is therefore needed for all people with diabetes.

THE NATURAL HISTORY OF THE DIABETIC FOOT

■ Neuropathy

Between 30 and 40% of diabetic patients in the United Kingdom will develop significant nerve damage during their diabetic lives because of suboptimal control of their diabetes.

Small fibre neuropathy

The earliest neuropathy modality to develop is small fibre neuropathy, with impaired pain and temperature perception. As the other sensory modalities might be intact, patients are often unaware

Fig. 1.1 This patient already had severe complications, including gangrene, when his diabetes was diagnosed. He felt no pain because of his neuropathy and could not see his foot problem because of retinopathy.

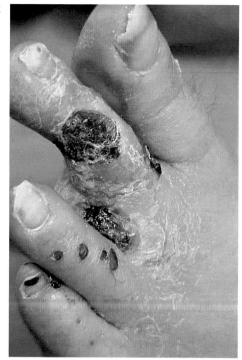

that there is a problem with their protective sensation. At this stage they are vulnerable to unperceived traumas, including burns, puncture wounds and other traumas, ulcers, and Charcot's osteoarthropathy.

Autonomic neuropathy
Patients who develop autonomic neuropathy might notice distended veins on the dorsum of the foot (known as 'Ward's sign' because it was first described by Professor John Ward of Sheffield). This is due to arteriovenous shunting and increased blood flow. The skin on the feet becomes dry. There is danger of skin fissures developing, which might eventually extend into the dermis and provide a portal of entry for infection (Fig. 1.2A).

Motor neuropathy

Patients might develop motor neuropathy, which is often associated with a typical deformity of raised arch and clawing of the toes (Fig 1.2B). This deformity leads to high pressure areas, which are susceptible to ulceration.

Large fibre neuropathy

Patients with small fibre neuropathy usually progress to develop large fibre neuropathy, with reduction of the sensations of touch,

Fig. 1.2 (A) Signs of neuropathy: lack of sweating leads to dry skin and fissures. (B) Signs of neuropathy: raised arch, claw toes and distended dorsal veins.

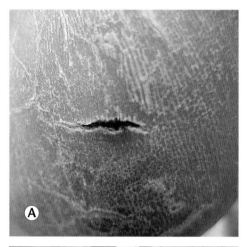

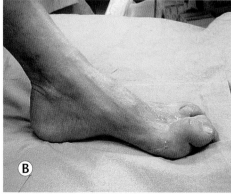

pressure, and proprioception (joint position sense). By now, patients are usually aware that there is a problem: that the feet and legs feel numb, or tingling, or as if there is a tight constricting band around them. Other patients complain that their feet feel cold, although, in fact, neuropathic feet are usually warm because the autonomic neuropathy leads to abnormal shunting of blood through the foot and increased blood flow. Some patients burn their feet by trying to warm them with hot water bottles or in front of the fire.

■ Callus and plantar neuropathic ulcers

Sites of high pressure on the soles of the foot with neuropathy are common and the skin can respond to pressure by developing callus. If the callus is not regularly removed by a podiatrist, the patient is likely to develop a neuropathic ulcer. Most neuropathic ulcers on the sole of the foot are associated with callus, and are painless, so patients have no direct incentive to seek help or to rest the foot.

■ Infection

If neuropathic ulcers become infected, patients might still feel no pain, fail to seek treatment and continue to walk. In these circum-stances a rapidly spreading infection can develop and destroy the foot within a few days.

■ 'Diabetic gangrene' (black toe)

Even though the blood supply to the neuropathic foot is good, a local infection can damage digital arteries and lead to a black toe in a foot with bounding pulses: this situation is often described as 'classic diabetic gangrene'.

■ Peripheral vascular disease

As the years of diabetic life go by, many patients with peripheral neuropathy will also develop peripheral vascular disease, which, in people with diabetes, has a particular delectation for the trifurcation of the tibial vessels at knee (popliteal) level. Most diabetic patients with peripheral vascular disease also have some degree of peripheral neuropathy, and it is only extremely rarely that podiatrists will encounter a purely ischaemic diabetic foot.

Once patients with neuropathy develop concurrent ischaemia they usually no longer develop heavy callus on the soles of the feet, because a good blood supply appears to be necessary for exuberant callus formation.

■ Intermittent claudication

Some neuroischaemic patients complain of intermittent claudication: however, if concurrent neuropathy is profound they will not claudicate.

■ Rest pain

Many diabetic patients with neuroischaemic feet do not complain of rest pain because neuropathy masks ischaemic pain.

■ Marginated ischaemic ulcers

Instead of the soles, it is the margins of neuroischaemic feet that are sites for ulceration. By the time they develop ulcers, many patients with peripheral vascular disease will also have cardiac or renal complications, both of which can lead to peripheral oedema, which renders the shoes tight, increases the risk of ulceration, and delays wound healing.

■ Wet and dry gangrene in the neuroischaemic foot

If ischaemic ulcers become infected the patient develops wet gangrene, or if the blood supply to the foot diminishes to a critical level, then the patient will develop dry gangrene.

■ Major amputation

If treatment is not successful, the patient may need a major amputation.

STATISTICS RELATING TO DIABETIC FOOT PROBLEMS

15% of people with diabetes will develop foot ulceration at some stage during their diabetic life and, at any one time, 5% of the diabetic population of the United Kingdom will have a foot ulcer. Many foot ulcers probably heal quickly and without complications, especially if the patient receives early care from a podiatrist. However, too many ulcers fail to heal, become indolent, develop infection, and come to amputation.

Eighty-five per cent of diabetic major amputations begin with a foot ulcer, and the common pathway to amputation involves infection entering the foot and leading to gangrene. The other 15% of major amputations will be due to rest pain, ischaemia that has destroyed the foot or an unstable Charcot joint.

Diabetic patients are between 15 and 25 times more likely to come to a major amputation than patients without diabetes.

A HOSTILE WORLD

On developing neuropathy or neuroischaemia, patients enter an unfamiliar and suddenly hostile world, where previously safe, everyday activities, like running for the bus or pottering barefoot around the house, can lead to serious foot problems. Trimming corns, applying proprietary remedies, and failing to seek timely expert help and advice can each cause a major disaster. Small breaks in the skin can develop a rapidly ascending infection and destroy the foot within a few days. Painless ulcers fail to heal and erode soft tissues and bone. Critical ischaemia leads to severe rest pain and necrosis.

IMPROVING OUTCOMES

Amputations are rarely inevitable, and podiatrists can often do a great deal to improve outcomes for diabetic foot patients by modifying risk factors, by providing preventive foot care and treatment of ulcers and, through education, making patients aware that they are at risk but that they are not helpless. This work should begin, whenever possible, before diabetic patients develop foot complications, so that good, sensible and practical foot care; regular foot inspections; and seeking expert help as soon as problems develop will become a diabetic way of life.

STAGING THE DIABETIC FOOT

When organizing risk factor modification it is useful for podiatrists to stage the diabetic foot as shown in Box 1.1.

These stages reflect the natural history of the diabetic foot, as described above. As the patient moves up through the stages, the need for specialized care increases, as does the risk of poor outcome, including healing failure and amputation. However, progression up

Box 1.1	**Staging the diabetic foot**
• Stage 1	the low risk foot
• Stage 2	the high risk foot
• Stage 3	the ulcerated foot
• Stage 4	the infected foot
• Stage 5	the necrotic foot
• Stage 6	the major amputation

the stages is not inevitable if problems are detected early, due precautions are taken, and treatment is offered and accepted. Further details of staging the diabetic foot are given in Chapter 3.

RATIONING PODIATRY

Good podiatric treatment can improve outcomes for diabetic foot patients. Because there is a shortage of podiatrists in the United Kingdom, and many other areas of the world, it is important to avoid unnecessary interventions and to refrain from offering regular podiatry to patients unless they have a clear need for it. To decide who needs podiatry it is necessary to do a risk assessment for each patient with diabetes.

KEY RISK FACTORS

The two most important risk factors for diabetic foot disease are:

● neuropathy
● ischaemia.

Neuropathy is the most significant risk factor of all because it is almost invariably present in every diabetic foot that gets into serious trouble.

SECONDARY RISK FACTORS

There are many further risk factors (which can be called secondary risk factors because they are of secondary importance). In themselves they might not be serious problems but they are important when found in combination with neuropathy and ischaemia because they greatly increase the likelihood of ulceration developing. The risks of ulceration accumulate in direct proportion to the number of risk factors present. Secondary risk factors include:

- unsuitable footwear
- iatrogenic lesions caused by unsuitable treatments
- self-treatment
- deformity
- swelling
- callus
- old age
- psychosocial problems
- diabetes complications
- going on holiday
- keeping a pet
- previous history of ulceration, minor or major amputation.

These risk factors are discussed in more detail below.

■ Neuropathy

Diabetic patients who develop peripheral neuropathy lose most of the warning signals that they are injuring themselves or developing an infection: a patient with neuropathy can be likened to a house without a smoke alarm.

'Belle indifference'

Lack of sensation also leads to a curious psychological problem where the part of the body affected by neuropathy no longer feels as if it belongs to the patient and might be resented, neglected or ignored. This indifferent state is often referred to as 'belle indifference'.

Podiatrists working in the field of diabetic foot care need to compensate for lack of protective pain sensation and *belle indifference* in their patients. To make neuropathic patients safer it is necessary to persuade them that they are at risk. This can sometimes be achieved by education. In addition to regular, sufficiently frequent, foot care delivered by a trained healthcare practitioner, patients with neuropathy benefit from regular and frequently updated education. However, no matter how well educated and careful patients with neuropathic feet might be, and how much preventive foot care they receive, they are always at risk of developing foot problems.

Good metabolic control can prevent or delay neuropathy

From the work of the multicentre diabetes control and complications trial (DCCT) in the USA and the United Kingdom prospective diabetes study (UKPDS) we know that the onset of neuropathy can be prevented or delayed by very tight (near normal) metabolic control. However, achieving near normal control of blood glucose is easier said than done. Many patients in the tight control arm of the DCCT who achieved near normal glycaemic control rapidly relapsed into less optimal states of control once they quit the study.

Dangers of late diagnosis

Many patients with type 2 diabetes face the problem of late diagnosis, and by the time they know that they have diabetes they already have profound neuropathy and other complications of diabetes. Indeed, some patients are only diagnosed diabetic when they present late with gangrene because neuropathy prevented them from feeling pain and retinopathy prevented them from seeing that their foot had become gangrenous. This is called 'eye foot syndrome'.

Aetiopathology of neuropathy

The aetiopathology of neuropathy is not entirely clear. Nerves in diabetic patients seem to be particularly susceptible to damage. There are several different theories as to why neuropathy arises: it might be accumulation of toxic substances within the nerve, or damage to the vasa nervorum (the small blood vessel supplying the nerve). Neuropathy might be caused by small vessel disease in the same way that the eyes and kidneys are damaged by small vessel disease. Thickening of the basement membrane of capillaries has been demonstrated in all of these sites: eyes, kidneys, and nerves. Studies by Professor John Ward's group in Sheffield, UK, also showed changes in the vasa nervorum in patients with painful neuropathy.

Treatment of neuropathy

There is no proven way of reversing neuropathy. However, even if neuropathy cannot be prevented or reversed, podiatrists and their patients should be aware that the effects of neuropathy on the foot can be modified with the interventions described below, which are discussed in greater detail in other chapters. The problems that arise in neuropathic feet are usually not due to neuropathy alone, but to unperceived injury or infection which is not detected or prevented because of neuropathy.

Strategies to reduce problems associated with neuropathy
Strategies include:

- Education programmes aimed at helping patients to perceive that they are at risk but also to believe that they are not helpless.
- Foot protection programmes offering suitable footwear; application of emollients to dry skin; and regular, sufficiently frequent podiatry to cut nails, remove callus, and detect and treat any other foot problems.
- Emergency services providing rapid access to help for patients in trouble.
- Specialist care for patients who develop the complications of the neuropathic foot (ulcers, gangrene, Charcot foot, neuropathic oedema) aiming at achieving rapid healing and preventing relapse.

Special education for patients with neuropathy
It is essential to teach patients with neuropathy that they are at risk of foot problems, to explain the effects of neuropathy on their perception of foot problems, and to enrol them in a trauma prevention foot protection programme. Above all, they must be taught that foot problems can be serious even though they do not hurt: that is the key message for them to take home. Unfortunately, it is a message that is frequently forgotten or not acted upon. Although it is easy to change knowledge it is not easy to change the beliefs and behaviour of consenting adults who have no pain to warn them of problems.

In patients without neuropathy, foot problems lead to severe pain or discomfort that cannot be ignored, and patients will seek help promptly. If a callus becomes too thick the patient will be forced to seek help from a podiatrist before ulceration develops. Neuropaths have no obvious warning of problems.

Most healthcare systems are 'symptom led' and rely on patients complaining. They often work well – except for patients who feel no pain, who are badly let down by modern health care.

Patients who enjoy reading should look at the wonderful book by the late Dr Paul Brand and Philip Yancy, *The Gift of Pain* (Zondervan Publishing House, Grand Rapids, Michigan, USA 1997), which gives patients and healthcare professionals fresh perspectives and valuable insights into the practical implications of having neuropathy.

Patients need to understand how easily neuropathic feet are damaged and the alarming speed at which diabetic foot problems can progress; a small, apparently clean ulcer can become infected and lead to extensive gangrene in the space of just 2 or 3 days.

However, there is a danger of instilling a sense of hopelessness in patients: they must be made aware of the risks but need to be reassured that they are not helpless and that with due care they will be able to lead a full and active life despite their neuropathy. Readers are referred to Chapter 9 for further details of educational strategies for people with diabetes, their families and their carers.

■ Ischaemia

Patients with ischaemic feet lose the ability to mount an adequate inflammatory response (which has a large vascular component) and thus have diminished ability to fight infection and to heal wounds. Neuropathy also affects the inflammatory response. Most patients with peripheral vascular disease will also have peripheral neuropathy and lack the usual signs and symptoms of vascular disease, such as intermittent claudication and rest pain, which are frequently reduced or absent in diabetic patients.

Feet with a combination of neuropathy and ischaemia are generally referred to as neuroischaemic feet. It is rare to see a purely ischaemic foot with no neuropathy in diabetes. The treatment of the purely ischaemic foot in diabetes is very similar to treatment for the neuro-ischaemic foot, differing only in the following ways:

- The need for pain control. Some purely ischaemic patients have agonizing rest pain
- The fact that debridement of the ischaemic foot might be impossible due to pain, and the patient will not allow the podiatrist to touch the feet.

Great care needs to be taken to avoid injury to neuroischaemic or ischaemic tissues when cutting and clearing nails and debriding callus or ulcers; underoperating should be the rule.

'Small vessel disease'

There is a great need for anatomical precision when podiatrists refer to 'small vessel disease' in the diabetic foot. At one time, all gangrene and much ulceration in the diabetic foot was deemed to be the result of 'small vessel disease'. Because small vessel disease was felt to be incurable, many patients with indolent ulcers or gangrene received above-knee amputations without further ado. A seminal paper by Frank Logerfo and colleagues in the *New England Journal of Medicine* in the 1980s showed that small vessel disease does not, in fact, play a significant part in the development of gangrene in the diabetic foot. Gangrene is usually due to infection or macrovascular disease. It is unfortunate that, in some centres, small vessel disease is still used as an excuse for lack of intervention and therapeutic nihilism. The term 'vascular disease', as used in this book, relates to macrovascular disease (arterial occlusive disease) affecting the leg arteries of diabetic foot patients with neuroischaemic feet.

Risk factors for development of peripheral vascular disease

Risk factors for vascular disease include poor glycaemic control, a high-fat diet, increased body mass index, lack of exercise, high blood pressure, and smoking. Outcomes can be improved with diet improvement, weight loss, and, where necessary, medication to improve the metabolic state, often including statins and low-dose aspirin. The onset of ischaemia can be prevented or delayed if hyperglycaemia, hypertension, and hyperlipidaemia are treated and patients avoid smoking (see Chapter 2).

Diagnosis of peripheral vascular disease

All patients should have their foot pulses palpated at initial screening. Those who present for examination with cold, pink, pulseless feet (Fig. 1.3) should have their ischaemia formally quantitated.

Strategies to protect patients with peripheral vascular disease

Those with a pressure index below 0.8 might need to be referred to the vascular team. Patients with intermittent claudication, rest pain, ischaemic ulcers or gangrene should definitely be given a referral to the multidisciplinary foot team (including a vascular specialist). Podiatrists should not forget that the 2004 NICE Guidelines on the management of the diabetic foot specify that diabetic foot patients with new pain, ulcers or gangrene should be seen very urgently (within 48 h).

All patients with a pressure index below 1 should receive special education with the emphasis on the importance of trauma avoid-

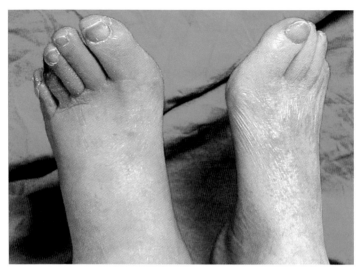

Fig. 1.3   A cold, pink, pulseless neuroischaemic foot.

ance and the early detection and treatment of any problems. The lower the pressure index, the worse the ischaemia, the worse the likely outcome, and the greater the need to prevent trauma and to report problems early.

Many patients with a very low pressure index do well so long as they can avoid injury to the feet and receive regular foot care. However, in severely ischaemic feet, even a tiny injury can lead to catastrophe, as the foot will be unable to mount an inflammatory response (with a large vascular component) sufficient to combat infection and achieve healing.

In diabetes, it is usually feet with a combination of neuropathy and ischaemia that come to major amputation, and patients with diabetic neuroischaemic feet develop problems earlier than non-diabetic patients with purely ischaemic feet. This is probably because patients without concurrent neuropathy will be almost immobile from intermittent claudication and rest pain by the time their feet are critically ischaemic, and their feet will be so painful that they will take great care to avoid injuring them. Many neuroischaemic diabetic patients never claudicate or feel rest pain and are more likely to walk and to injure their feet.

Injudicious warming of cold feet, barefoot walking, and unsuitable footwear commonly cause problems in the neuroischaemic foot.

■ Poor footwear

Unsuitable shoes and socks are a frequent cause of ulceration in both neuropathic and neuroischaemic feet by virtue of the following factors:

- size
- style
- design
- construction
- state of wear.

In addition, high-risk patients who do not wear shoes and walk barefoot are very vulnerable to injury (see Chapter 4 for further details of appropriate offloading).

Size and style

If the shoes are too narrow, shallow or short, the patient will be at risk of pressure lesions over the toes and apices of the toes, and overloading of plantar sites. If the shoes are too long or loose, especially if there is no proper fastening mechanism, then frictional forces can cause blisters or calluses.

The feet should be measured towards the end of the day because feet swell during the course of the day and it is important for any oedema to be accommodated. They should be measured with the patient in a standing position because the weight-bearing foot is longer and wider than the offloaded foot.

Patients with neuropathy should be warned that the previous familiar sensation of feeling the shoes on the feet will be lost and that if they can still feel their shoes on their feet this is probably because the shoes are too tight. It is a good idea to make a paper tracing of the standing foot and see whether it fits easily into the new shoe.

When fitting shoes for the high-risk diabetic foot the following points are important:

- A 'dead space' of at least 1.5 cm should be present between the tips of the toes and the toe box of the shoe when the patient is standing.

- The shoe should avoid pressure points over the toes or on the margins of the foot.
- The heel cup should fit snugly around the heel.
- The shoes should fasten with a lace or strap to prevent friction.
- The heel should be below 5 cm in height.
- The sole of the shoe should be thick enough to protect the foot from puncture wounds.

Patients with neuropathy and callus or previous history of ulceration might need a specially designed insole, which will often need to be accommodated in a bespoke shoe. When fitting shoes, the need to accommodate insoles and orthotics should always be taken into account.

Neuroischaemic feet need to have the vulnerable margins protected in extra-depth, wide-fitting shoes.

Sports shoes are useful for people with diabetes whose feet are not severely deformed.

Even if a new pair of shoes appears to be a perfect fit, they should not be worn for long periods at first and, when the shoes are removed, the feet should be checked for red marks or hot spots, which might indicate that the new shoes are too tight.

State of wear

Once the shoes are in regular current use, the state of wear of shoes should be regularly monitored. The upper part of the shoe might stretch so that the laces are no longer effective and a tongue pad might be needed to prevent friction. Linings can become stiff or ruckled, foreign bodies might be dropped into the shoes, and nails or other sharp objects can penetrate thin soles. Patients with neuropathy or neuroischaemia should always shake out their shoes before they put them on, and run a hand around the inside of the shoe to detect rough places. Patients with poor eyesight or neuropathic hands will need help checking their shoes, in the same way that they will need help with their daily foot check. Eternal vigilance is the only key to safety for patients with neuropathy.

There are strong and subtle social and emotional pressures on people to wear unsuitable shoes. The great Jazz singer, Ella Fitzgerald, had type 2 diabetes, underwent bilateral major amputations and announced that she had lost her legs through wearing 'pointy toed shoes'.

Pressures on patients to wear unsuitable shoes need to be countered with education. However, it is cruel to tell a young, fashion-conscious patient that she must wear 'Granny' shoes for the rest of her life, or a diabetic child that he should never go barefoot. Compromise is often needed. Many a pair of bespoke hospital shoes has been made at great expense only to end up in the back of the patient's wardrobe, and prescribing shoes is useless if patients do not wear them.

The Sex Life of the Foot and Shoe by William A Rossi (Routledge & Kegan Paul, London 1977) is highly recommended to readers because it gives insight into the psychological aspects of footwear choice.

Holes in shoes or socks, lumpy darns, and wearing damp footwear and hose can also cause foot ulcers.

Iatrogenic lesions

Some severe injuries to the diabetic foot can be iatrogenic in nature, being the result of treatment offered for diabetic foot problems by podiatrists. Examples are infected rubs within total contact casts, application of salicylic-acid-based corn and callus remedies causing severe chemical burns, and injudicious operating on ischaemic feet leading to spreading tissue necrosis. Many treatments that are suitable for non-diabetic feet can cause severe problems if applied to the high-risk diabetic foot. As the diabetic foot develops risk factors, it is necessary for the podiatrist to reconsider every aspect of treatment.

Self-treatment

Patients who attempt self-diagnosis or self-treatment are very much at risk, and footcare education programmes should warn patients to seek help from a properly qualified healthcare professional if foot problems arise or they need advice about foot care. Foot spas can cause burns and blisters, and patients' attempts to cut their own toenails in the presence of poor vision or ischaemia are common causes of problems. 'Bathroom surgery', where patients cut their own corns and calluses, or debride ulcers themselves, should be avoided. Self-treatment with proprietary corn cures can lead to severe damage.

Deformity

This might be temporary or permanent, congenital or acquired. Deformities can be the result of diabetes or unrelated to the diabetes.

Examples of diabetic foot swelling causing temporary deformity include the 'sausage toe' presentation of osteomyelitis, fracture, dislocation, bursitis and soft tissue infection. Reorganization of tissues, as in wound contracture, may lead to permanent deformity. The most common diabetic foot deformities include:

- the 'classical' neuropathic foot deformity consisting of high arch and clawing of the toes
- foot drop
- claw, hammer and mallet toes
- hallux rigidus or limitus
- plantar flexion of the foot and other manifestations of limited joint mobility
- lack of fibro fatty padding.

Deformity can be fixed or flexible, involving bone or joint or soft tissue, and can often be due to soft tissue contracture or depletion.

Charcot foot deformity
Late diagnosis and suboptimal management of Charcot's osteo-arthropathy can lead to deformity, including:

- medial convexity
- rocker bottom
- flail ankle.

For details of Charcot's osteoarthropathy, see Chapter 7.

Prophylactic surgery for deformed feet
Podiatrists with surgical training might wish to consider the possibility of undertaking prophylactic surgery to prevent future problems: other podiatrists may consider referral of the patient on to them for surgery. However, if the foot is severely neuropathic or neuroischaemic, surgery can be contraindicated. Elective surgery to the neuropathic foot can occasionally trigger a Charcot's osteo-arthropathy: surgery to the neuroischaemic foot may not heal, and rates of postoperative infection are higher in diabetic patients than in those without diabetes.

Palliative care of deformity
Special footwear and orthotics will often accommodate deformity successfully and compensate for biomechanical abnormality, as

when a shoe with a built in rocker sole is provided to compensate for overloading at toe off caused by a hallux rigidus (for further details of offloading techniques, see Chapter 4).

■ Swelling

There are many different causes of unilateral or bilateral oedema. Testing for pitting oedema (Fig. 1.4) is performed as follows: the podiatrist presses the oedematous area gently but firmly, to express fluid from the tissues. The pressure is maintained for 10 seconds. When the finger is removed, a pit or depression is seen on the site subjected to pressure. The worse the oedema, the deeper the pit will be.

Patients who present to the podiatrist with severe leg oedema and shortage of breath need rapid medical review by a physician. New onset of oedema in a patient with distended neck veins and a visible jugular venous pulse indicates that the patient is in congestive heart failure and a physician should see the patient urgently.

Podiatrists should remember that myocardial infarction is common in neuroischaemic patients and is sometimes painless because of neuropathy ('silent infarction'). A patient with myocardial infarc-

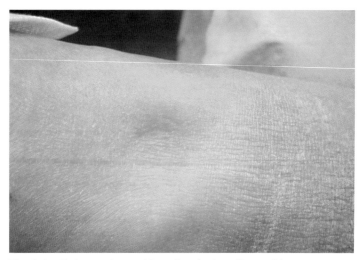

Fig. 1.4   Pitting oedema: this patient had cardiac problems.

tion complaining only of pain in his jaw was recently seen by the author. Chest pain in a diabetic patient is a clinical emergency.

Common causes of unilateral oedema

Causes of unilateral oedema include:

- Charcot's osteoarthropathy
- fracture or soft tissue injury
- infection
- deep vein thrombosis
- gout
- malignancy.

Causes of bilateral oedema

These include:

- Cardiac insufficiency
- Renal insufficiency
- Neuropathic oedema
- Venous insufficiency.

Conservative/palliative management of oedema

A pair of roomy shoes with adjustable fastenings is necessary to accommodate oedema. The podiatrist should refer the patient to the physician for treatment of causative factors such as cardiac problems or renal problems.

Neuropathic oedema

Very rarely the oedema is neuropathic oedema, which can be successfully treated with ephedrine, an old fashioned Chinese drug, which constricts blood vessels. Ephedrine is remarkably effective: one of the author's patients has been taking it for over 20 years without side effects.

Support stockings

If the patient has venous insufficiency then, in the absence of ischaemia, support stockings can be helpful. However, the nail sulci of patients in support stockings or tights are vulnerable, as pressure in this area from the hose can lead to onychocryptosis or ulcers. If the patient is ischaemic and the pressure index is below 0.8 then support stockings are contraindicated. Four-layer compression bandaging is unsuitable for ischaemic patients with venous ulceration: lesser degrees of compression might sometimes be possible.

The patient should take care to avoid injuries to oedematous tissues. (One of the author's patients went to great lengths to protect himself and wore old fashioned gaiters to prevent injury to his shins.)

■ Callus

Callus is one of the most important risk factors of all because it gives forewarning of an impending neuropathic ulcer. Heavy callus containing speckles of blood is an indicator of unacceptably high plantar pressures or other dangerously abnormal mechanical forces, and of incipient breakdown of the skin. This is a valuable marker for a shoe problem of style or fit.

There is a three-fold approach to the management of callus on the intact foot involving one or more of the following:

- prevention
- removal
- application of emollient.

Prevention

Callus can often be prevented from forming, by using suitable devices such as footwear, insoles, felt padding or orthotics to reduce the abnormal mechanical forces leading to inflammation and callus formation.

Removal

Sharp debridement with a scalpel is necessary when prevention fails and it is not possible to stop callus forming. It is essential that people with diabetes perceive callus on the foot as a potentially serious problem, which will lead to ulceration without treatment, and seek help from podiatrists. Patients and their families need to inspect callus for small black or brown speckles, which are the danger sign that, without prompt removal of callus, an ulcer will develop.

Application of emollient

Callus should be kept well moistened with an emollient such as E45 cream (or Calmurid for recalcitrant cases) as otherwise it can develop fissures. If fissures penetrate to the dermis then ulceration frequently results.

Caustics

The author has never recommended use of silver nitrate or ferric chloride to slow down callus formation in the high-risk diabetic foot because these products cause discoloration that might mask signs of infection or necrosis.

Adjunctive self-care by the patient to remove callus

Patients with good vision and minimal neuropathy can be advised to use a pumice stone to rub down callus gently, thus preventing accumulation of sufficient thickness to cause problems.

Removal of callus by the podiatrist

In the neuropathic foot, callus is often thick and exuberant and is removed with a scalpel. The podiatrist holds the scalpel between thumb and fingers (Fig 1.5) and strokes the blade through the callus with a sideways, rather than a downwards, movement to remove a thin slicket (little slice) of callus with each stroke of the scalpel. It is a mistake to try and remove too much callus with each stroke, or to saw at the foot as if carving a joint: each stroke of the scalpel should be clean and distinct from the strokes before and after it. The surface from the whole plaque should be removed to a uniform depth before removing the deeper areas, beginning at the centre of the plaque and working outwards. The podiatrist will need to use a combination of visual and tactile clues to guide her and tell her when to stop.

The deepest callus will usually be towards the centre of the plaque. If it is difficult to distinguish between what is callus and

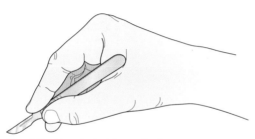

Fig. 1.5   How to hold a scalpel.

what is skin, then the plaque of callus can be moistened with surgical spirit, which will make deeper areas look more distinct.

Having removed most of the plaque there may be discrete areas that are deeper and which need to be dissected out. The operator should lift a piece of callus, grip it with forceps, apply gentle traction, and start to dissect out the deeper area; this might be in a ridge formation or a small discrete area constituting a corn. The operator might want to dissect them out without applying traction but the author has usually found that the application of traction through forceps improves precision.

The thumb and forefinger of the other hand, when not occupied with forceps, are used to stretch the skin (applying skin tension), which renders removal of callus easier, avoids uneven removal, immobilizes the area being worked on, and makes it less likely that the patient will be inadvertently injured.

Ischaemic callus

Most severely ischaemic feet do not develop callus, but where ischaemic callus is present it is usually found in thin, glassy plaques. The thickness of the plaques is extremely deceptive, and the blade of the scalpel is prone to slip and skid on the glassy consistency, so great care needs to be taken to avoid cutting the patient.

Callus around ulcers

Callus often forms around neuropathic ulcers and is a physical barrier to the growth of new epithelium from the edges of the ulcer. Further-more, callus can sometimes seal off the ulcer cavity, preventing drainage, following which the foot deteriorates rapidly. It is difficult to ascertain the true dimensions of an ulcer unless all associated callus is debrided away. A halo of thick callus around a neuropathic ulcer transmits high pressure to the underlying tissues, which might lead to enlargement of the ulcer. For all these reasons it is best to remove callus from around neuropathic ulcers.

Ischaemic ulcers can also develop a halo of callus, but the callus is usually very thin and glassy. The operator should beware of over-operating on ischaemic callus because it is very easy to cut the patient if the blade of the scalpel skids on the glassy callus.

Patients who have been on a beach holiday might present with callus which is impregnated with sand. Often the first sign that there is a problem is when the blade of the scalpel hits a particle and loses its edge immediately; this is often accompanied by a screeching sound-effect like chalk on a blackboard.

Studies have been performed with collagen and silicone implants to augment fibro fatty padding and thus reduce callus formation, but neither technique is widely used.

■ Old age

Problems found in elderly diabetic patients include neuropathy, which is present in many elderly people, whether diabetic or not. Readers are referred to the age-corrected tables of Bloom and Sonksen (Stephen Bloom was a medical student at St Thomas' Hospital who, for a project, measured vibration perception threshold in hundreds of normal subjects and ascertained mean vibration perception thresholds for different age groups, thus producing data for one of the most widely quoted papers in the field of neuropathy and the diabetic foot, and achieving a publication in the *British Medical Journal* even before he qualified as a doctor.)

Some elderly diabetic patients lack any perception that their problems can be helped by the podiatrist. Many have a fierce determination to maintain their independence. When the author began working for Camberwell Health Authority, some elderly patients were reluctant to come into St Giles Hospital, a local hospital, because the buildings were the former workhouse. Other elderly patients have physical difficulties in accessing care and getting to the hospital or clinic but are reluctant to admit that they have problems. Social services departments can sometimes help, as can rallying the family, friends and neighbours to support the patient.

Concurrent mental illness

Acute bipolar disorder and schizophrenia are particularly difficult problems. Some patients are abusive to staff and may be denied treatment or access to clinics. Especially when coupled with neuropathy, mental illness is a great barrier to care. Depression leads to apathy and indifference to foot problems, and when neuropathy is present it is very easy for patients to ignore their feet.

Many patients with mental illness are incapable of enjoying life, and feel hopeless, hapless and helpless.

Extra help will be needed and should be enlisted from families, friends and carers. Podiatrists should be sympathetic to these patients, who often behave 'badly' only because of their illness and will respond to kindness and sympathy. Most patients with serious mental illness have a special social worker, who should be contacted and involved in clinical decisions.

▦ Patients with intellectual deficit

Patients with intellectual deficit may be unable to look after their feet adequately, to detect problems or to understand the need for treatment. Families and carers should be involved in their foot care and asked to bring them to the clinic regularly and check their feet for problems between appointments.

▦ Irregular attendances

Reasons for failed appointments should be ascertained: sometimes there are good reasons for patients not keeping their appointments or failing to arrive on time.

▦ Social isolation

This is a particular problem for elderly frail patients with neuropathy and poor vision. In these circumstances, podiatrists often need to depend on the patient's family to keep an eye on the feet and make contact in emergency on the patient's behalf if problems arise. In the absence of family and friends, there may be a need for more frequent appointments to ensure that problems are caught early.

▦ Poverty

Poverty and social deprivation can have profound effects on diabetes and the diabetic foot. Inadequate heating in winter puts the feet at risk. Associated problems include cheap, worn-out shoes, inadequate diet, walking long distances because of the expense of transport, low health expectations, lack of adequate heating and hot water, cold and damp living conditions and unreliable lifts in high rise flats. A study by Professor John Ward has linked diabetic foot problems and social deprivation.

One of the author's patients was unable to take part in a clinical trial because he had no refrigerator at home in which to keep the trial product. Instead, he had an old fashioned 'meat safe' (a cupboard screened with perforated zinc sheeting against flies). He was unable to rest his ulcerated foot sufficiently because he had to go out every day to shop for perishable food items.

▥ Poor accommodation

Cold, damp, draughty accommodation, many flights of stairs, and lifts that break-down frequently are all bad for the diabetic foot. Some patients benefit from rehousing and letters of support on medical grounds can be written by the podiatrist, who can also act as a patient's advocate.

▥ Ignorance

All diabetic patients need to know how to look after their feet, what are suitable shoes for them, and what to do and where to go if they develop a problem. Education can modify behaviour and reduce the incidence of diabetic foot problems.

It is disconcerting to treat a frail, high-risk diabetic patient who has no idea what medication he is taking, what other health problems he has, whether he is allergic to penicillin, how long he has had diabetes or which hospitals he is attending. It is worrying to talk to a patient who, only a few months ago, suffered a severe foot infection with loss of several toes, spent weeks in hospital and who has a long history of foot problems, and to realize that he has forgotten all the careful education he received about the dangers of neuropathy, that foot problems can be serious without being painful, and that he should always seek same-day treatment in an emergency. Ignorance is an important risk factor, and needs to be countered by frequent education, pitched at the correct level for the patient, and an open door policy for patients in trouble, whose families and other carers should be alerted to the difficulty.

▥ Barefoot walking

It is not necessary to instruct all people with diabetes never to walk bare foot, just as it is not necessary for the general population to avoid ever walking without shoes. However, in the presence of neuropathy and ischaemia, patients should be specifically advised to refrain from barefoot walking. Stubbed toes, puncture wounds, and other traumas are commonly seen in patients who fail to follow this advice. However, some patients may be subjected to pressure to walk barefoot because of cultural or religious reasons. There is a large immigrant population in the UK from the Indian subcontinent, who traditionally go barefoot round the house and when they go to the temple. The social pressures on them to conform are considerable and a blanket ban on barefoot walking might may not be practical.

However, such patients should be advised to take great care to clear up spilt or broken substances immediately, to check their feet on a daily basis for injuries, and to report problems early.

■ Employment
Some occupations are particularly hazardous for people at high risk of developing diabetic foot problems. If possible, jobs entailing long hours of standing or walking, or the need to wear unsuitable foot-wear, are best avoided.

■ Pulling and picking off pieces of skin or nail (Fig. 1.6)
This is a difficult habit to break, and many serious infections begin when the feet are picked and the skin is broken. Keeping the shoes and socks on except when in bed or in the bath, and applying emollient to tempting pieces of projecting dry skin might be helpful.

■ Eye problems
Poor vision leads to failure to detect foot problems early and increased likelihood of trauma. The friends and families of patients with eye problems should be asked to help the patient.

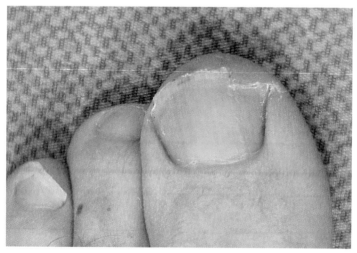

Fig. 1.6   A neglected foot. This patient does not cut his toenails but picks at them instead.

■ Hyperglycaemia

Patients with hyperglycaemia are prone to develop complications, and more likely to develop infection. Help will be needed from other members of the team, including the physician and the diabetes specialist nurse.

■ Hypoglycaemia

Traumatic lesions are common in patients who have suffered a hypoglycaemic episode. Periods of unconsciousness can lead to pressure lesions, burns and falls. Some patients who have been 'hypo' develop blisters on the feet.

Patients in whom hyperglycaemia or hypoglycaemia are recurring problems should be seen by the diabetes specialist nurse and diabetologist.

■ Postural hypotension and poor proprioception

Patients with neuropathy often develop postural hypotension and are very unsteady when they rise from a sitting or lying position and therefore risk falls. If this is a problem, patients should be taught to rise slowly and gradually, not to start walking until they feel steady and to report the problem to the diabetic physician. Patients with sensory neuropathy often lack joint positional sense and are also prone to injury. A stick or crutch might be helpful.

■ Holidays

Foot problems are common among diabetic foot patients who go on holiday. Holiday foot problems are often caused by walking barefoot on the beach or in the sea or in unfamiliar hotel or apartment accommodation, shoe rubs, and walking too far at airports.

All patients should be advised to take a simple first aid kit on holiday. People with very high-risk feet or current problems such as ulceration can be given the contact number of a local Health Professions Council (HPC) registered podiatrist: details are available from the Society of Chiropodists and Podiatrists (see Appendix).

■ Keeping a pet

Hairs from certain breeds of dog are stiff with sharp ends and can work themselves under human skin and cause inflammation (Fig. 1.7).

Dr David Armstrong, an American podiatrist, has described the case of a pet dog that, on two separate occasions nibbled his dozing

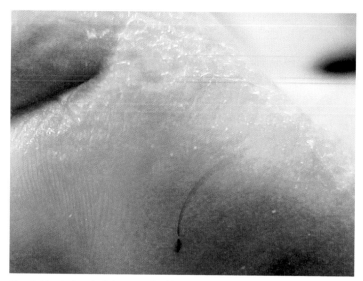

Fig. 1.7   A dog hair has worked its way under the skin.

owner's ulcerated foot causing considerable tissue defects. The saliva of carnivorous animals contains microorganisms that can lead to severe infection if pet dogs and cats are allowed to lick ulcers or wounds.

However, pet keeping can also have positive effects. Dr Paul Brand, who worked with neuropathic patients in India, always advised them to keep a cat in the house to keep the rats down and thus avoid rat bites to insensitive toes.

The author has never forgotten an encounter with a charming Labrador guide dog, brought to clinic by his blind owner, who, following an extensive debridement of callus and necrotic tissue, kindly licked the floor clean while her back was turned.

■ Previous history of ulceration, minor or major amputation

Relapse is frequent in diabetic foot patients. Both neuropathy and ischaemia are usually bilateral. A diabetic patient who has lost one leg is at great risk of losing the remaining one. Follow-up studies of diabetic major amputees have shown that within 3 years half will have died and that of the survivors, half will have lost the remaining leg. However, with well-organized foot care in a multidisciplinary diabetic foot clinic, it is possible to improve outcomes and reduce morbidity and mortality in diabetic major amputees.

A FOOT THAT IS ALMOST GUARANTEED TO GET INTO TROUBLE

There are, then, many different risk factors and reasons why diabetic feet go wrong, as discussed above. If you were setting out to draw up a blueprint for a foot that is almost guaranteed to get into trouble you could hardly do better than to design a model of a diabetic foot, with reduced ability to perceive pain, to heal and to fight infection, and which is pounded against the ground many times a day!

Some diabetic foot problems are beyond the scope of podiatrists, or anybody, to deal with. Some can only be solved if large amounts of money are available. However, most patients can be helped by an enthusiastic and dedicated podiatrist.

Case study

A patient, who is now 35 years old, was diagnosed with type 1 diabetes at the age of nine. She had a stormy adolescence, resisted all attempts to help her control and monitor her diabetes, and failed to attend regularly at the diabetic department. Aged 19 she awoke one morning to find that she had gone blind overnight, due to bilateral massive bleeds into the vitreous humour. She never regained her vision and was registered blind. In her twenties she married and had a son. She was a frequent foot clinic attender with neuropathic ulcers. At the age of 30 she developed end-stage renal failure, was given haemodialysis, and was then offered a combined kidney pancreas transplant. She is now off insulin, and her young son checks her feet every day and brings her to the clinic if problems arise between appointments.

FOOT PROTECTION PROGRAMMES

A large study in the United Kingdom by the British podiatrist McCabe and colleagues showed significant reduction of amputations in patients offered education and regular podiatry. Similar work, as yet unpublished, led by Drs Margreet van Putten and Nicholaas Schaper in the Netherlands, shows that a podiatry and foot protection programme can improve outcomes in high-risk diabetic patients.

The author established a foot protection programme in 1987 as part of a care plan for patients with diabetes and a kidney transplant. The patients were screened for neuropathy and ischaemia, their shoes were removed and feet checked every month without fail at their regular renal clinic attendance, and many problems were caught early. Outcomes in this group of patients were as good as for diabetic foot patients without renal transplants and gangrene and major amputations were reduced.

EMERGENCY SERVICES

Despite the best of care and attention, things can and will go wrong for people who lack protective pain sensation. No matter how careful patients are, it is impossible to protect the feet all of the time when pain sensation is lacking. An example of this is given in the following case study.

Case study

A 47-year-old man with type 2 diabetes and profound neuropathy was very careful of his feet. He checked them every day, wore special shoes, and attended the foot clinic regularly. He spent a night in a hotel in Scotland and burnt his feet badly on a hot water pipe running along the wall by his bed. He was woken in the night by a smell of roasting meat, and found a third-degree burn on the sole of his foot.

■ The emergency foot clinic

All patients who have neuropathy or neuroischaemia and develop a foot problem should have guaranteed same-day access to an emergency foot clinic so that treatment of the problem can be started without delay. The worst feet present after delays of several days or even weeks and if the problem is Charcot's osteoarthropathy or infection then irreparable damage might already have occurred. The earlier a patient is seen the sooner treatment can be started.

Emergency foot clinics can be manned by podiatrists and run concurrently with routine foot clinics.

A survey compared outcomes in patients who attended a diabetic foot clinic in emergency with outcomes in patients who had detected a foot problem but waited for treatment until their next routine appointment. The patients who attended in emergency did significantly better.

Many diabetic foot patients are elderly and frail: the mean age of the high-risk patients attending the foot clinic at King's College Hospital is 59 years, and similar mean ages are reported in studies from other foot clinics. It is important to make arrangements for patients to be brought to the clinic urgently on the same day that they find a problem. As ambulance services often need to be pre-booked several days in advance, accessing the clinic in emergency can be a problem and family, friends or relatives might need to take responsibility for bringing the patient in.

WORKING BACKWARDS

Risk factors might be perceived only after a problem has developed. It is a good exercise, whenever a podiatrist encounters a diabetic foot gone wrong, for the podiatrist to try to work backwards and discover what happened to that foot to set it on the road to amputation. It is important to know the timescale, and why steps that would have succeeded in protecting the foot were not taken. Podiatrists can only hope to prevent diabetic foot catastrophes in the future if they understand why they occurred in the past and learn lessons from history. The late Roger Peccararo, an American diabetic physician, helped to find causes of amputation when he and his colleagues sought out and described pathways to amputation.

Some community-based podiatrists appear to underestimate the dangers faced by diabetic foot patients. It should never be forgotten that many amputations probably begin with an apparently minor problem that is neglected or given inappropriate care.

FOOT PROTECTION PROGRAMMES FOR DIABETIC PATIENTS

▦ The newly diagnosed patient

Every diabetic patient needs to know the basic information about footcare, footwear, danger signs, first aid, and details of how to access help in order to be safe from present or future foot catastrophes.

However, in the very early days of a patient's diabetic life, he will be inundated with education and is in danger of information overload, when the brain is unable to process the quantity of education offered. For this reason, whenever possible, footcare education should be delayed for a few weeks, while metabolic control is addressed. However, every newly diagnosed diabetic should have his feet quickly checked for active problems, to ensure that ulcers and infections receive treatment, and no diabetic patient should ever be under the delusion that his diabetes is 'mild' or that his feet are not important.

▦ The stage 1 patient (without any foot complications)

Stage 1 patients are low risk. However, activities such as screening for risk factors that can give rise to foot problems, and offering preventive foot care to prevent or delay the onset of future problems, are very important parts of the role of the podiatrist in stage 1 diabetic foot care. Most of this work can be performed by podiatrists working for primary care trusts in the community.

Management aims

- To help patients to achieve good metabolic control.
- To educate patients in good footcare and footwear.
- To establish the need for annual review for all patients with diabetes when their feet will be reassessed.
- To explain why footcare is important to people with diabetes and make patients perceive that they are at long-term risk.

▦ The stage 2 patient (high risk but without current ulceration)

In theory, well-educated patients with neuropathy and ischaemia can be protected from many foot problems and managed routinely in the community. In practice, however, high-risk diabetic foot patients, especially if they are elderly, frail, impoverished and socially isolated, cannot always be depended on to do all the things that are necessary to keep their feet in a good state. They should not be judged too harshly when they fail to prevent problems, and often benefit from extra support and encouragement, and education that is specifically geared to their situation.

Management aims

- To make patients aware that they are at risk and to enable them to modify their life-style to avoid trauma and ulcers.
- To educate patients in foot care, foot wear, early detection of problems and the need for rapid help.
- To sharp-debride callus regularly and reduce its development with pressure-relieving devices.
- To accommodate deformity and oedema in suitable shoes.

▥ The stage 3 foot (with ulceration)

Once the patient has developed an ulcer (Fig. 1.8) this should be regarded as a pivotal event on the road to amputation; 85% of major amputations begin with a foot ulcer. Although many diabetic foot ulcers heal quickly, their propensity to destroy the foot should always be remembered. The NICE guidelines on diabetic foot care state that any diabetic patient with a new foot ulcer should be assessed by an expert foot team. Any ulcer that is not healing well within 4 weeks of first presentation, or which presents late, should be referred as soon as possible to a hospital-based multidisciplinary foot team with access to vascular investigations and surgery. It should never be forgotten that foot ulcer, past or present, is a major risk factor for amputation.

Management aims

- To heal the ulcer as quickly as possible.
- To prevent the ulcer from recurring.
- To prevent other ulcers from developing.
- To prevent all ulcers from deteriorating.
- To detect any deterioration as soon as possible.
- To ensure that after healing patients are followed up in a foot protection programme.

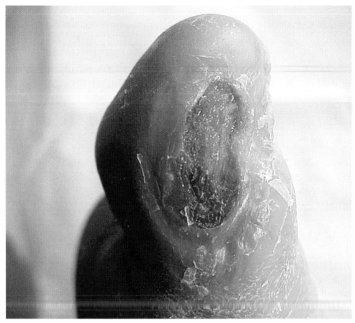

Fig. 1.8   An ischaemic ulcer on the medial border of the hallux needs care from a multidisciplinary team.

● To educate patients in ulcer care, signs of deterioration and the need for effective offloading.

■ The stage 4 foot (with infection)

Infection is a great destroyer of the diabetic foot and signs and symptoms of infection are often absent or diminished in people with diabetes. At present there is no easy way of differentiating between slight infections, which will clear quickly, and apparently slight infections that will suddenly become invasive and rapidly destroy tissue. It is important to remember that infection is almost always involved in the final common pathway to amputation and to believe that infection is a major risk factor for amputation. The patient with foot infection has a potentially limb-threatening condition. Podiatrists encountering infected diabetic feet should not work in isolation and the patient is ideally managed in a multi-disciplinary foot clinic with an experienced physician and surgeon on call.

Management aims

- To clear the infection as quickly as possible with rapid aggressive treatment (debridement, drainage, antibiotics).
- To prevent deterioration.
- To detect any deterioration as soon as possible.

■ The stage 5 foot (with necrosis)

Necrosis is always a very serious problem. It can be wet, when it is due to infection, or dry, when it is the result of peripheral vascular disease (or has been previously wet but responded to treatment with antibiotics).

Diabetic feet do not tolerate necrosis well. The problem is frequently more extensive than surface appearances indicate (iceberg foot). Necrotic feet should never be treated by isolated podiatrists: a multidisciplinary team approach is always necessary (Fig 1.9).

Fig.1.9 This ischaemic patient with dry necrosis needs urgent treatment. Angioplasty or bypass will speed healing of the foot. Assessment by the vascular team should be arranged without delay.

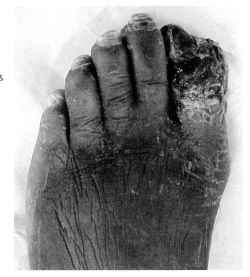

Management aims

- To control infection associated with wet necrosis and debride away wet necrotic tissue.
- To control peripheral vascular disease associated with dry necrosis and either amputate necrotic tissue or allow 'autoamputation' to take place.
- To offer podiatric debridement and dressings as appropriate until healing has occurred.
- To monitor the necrotic foot regularly to detect any deterioration as quickly as possible.

▓ The stage 6 foot (major amputation)

When a patient has undergone a major amputation the remaining foot is at great risk.

Management aims

- To rehabilitate patients as well as possible.
- To heal the stump.
- To offer regular assessment and preventive foot care for the remaining foot.

2 Reducing the impact of diabetic foot complications with good metabolic control

I have more flesh than another man, and therefore more frailty.

William Shakespeare, Henry IV Part I. II. I. 187

To treat diabetic foot problems successfully, podiatrists need to understand:

- The nature of diabetes.
- How it is diagnosed, treated and monitored, including:
  - diabetic diets
  - exercise
  - medication
  - management of diabetes during periods of acute illness.
- The nature of diabetic complications.
- How complications are prevented and treated.
- The roles of other members of the multidisciplinary diabetes team.

Although podiatrists cannot expect to become experts in every aspect of diabetes management, they should, if working with people with diabetes, be able to impart simple, up-to-date advice on most areas of diabetes care, in addition to filling the podiatrist's traditional role of giving advice on foot care and offering preventive foot care, foot treatments and education.

Knowledge of diabetes management makes it easier for podiatrists to communicate with other members of the diabetes team.

It is important that messages imparted by different members of the team about all aspects of diabetes management are consistent.

The other (non-podiatric) members of the diabetes team also need to be well informed about footwear and foot care, and it is part of the role of the podiatrist to educate other healthcare professionals in these areas.

Many people with diabetes are not managed in hospitals but in the community, often in diabetic clinics run by general practitioners and practice nurses. Community diabetes clinics should have access to podiatry services and should screen patients regularly (at least, on an annual basis) for foot problems.

Diabetic foot patients at stages 1 (low risk) and 2 (high risk) can be treated in the community, but this is not optimal care for patients at stages 3 (ulcer), 4 (infection) and 5 (necrosis) unless the community podiatrist works together with the practice nurse and general practitioner within a 'shared care' programme where the community team has support from the hospital team.

- The higher the foot stage, the more complicated it will be to achieve metabolic control.
- Hospital clinics usually have rapid access to investigations, interventions and hospital beds, which may not be quickly available in primary care.

WHAT IS DIABETES MELLITUS?

People develop diabetes when:

- The pancreas does not make any insulin.
- The pancreas does not make enough insulin.
- The cells in the muscles, liver, and fat do not use insulin properly: this is called insulin resistance.

There might be a combination of insufficient insulin and insulin resistance. When there is complete or partial lack of insulin, or insulin resistance, or both, then diabetes is diagnosed

Insulin is produced in the beta cells of the Islets of Langherhans in the pancreas. Its function is to enable the body tissues to take up glucose. As a result of diabetes, the amount of glucose in the blood increases above normal limits (hyperglycaemia) and the cells are starved of energy. Over many years, hyperglycaemia damages nerves and blood vessels, resulting in diabetic complications.

TYPES OF DIABETES AND MODERN NOMENCLATURE

■ Prediabetes

In the clinical state of 'prediabetes' (which was previously called 'impaired glucose tolerance'), blood glucose levels are higher than normal but not high enough for diabetes to be diagnosed. Many people with prediabetes go on to develop type 2 diabetes within 10 years; prediabetes also increases the risk of heart disease and stroke. However, if people with prediabetes manage to lose weight and take sufficient exercise, then they might be able to delay or prevent the onset of type 2 diabetes. Overweight people with diabetes who manage to lose weight with diet and exercise often find their diabetes far easier to control and can sometimes reduce or stop taking insulin or oral hypoglycaemic agents.

■ Type 1 diabetes mellitus

In type 1 diabetes, there is lack of insulin because the immune system has destroyed the insulin-manufacturing beta cells in the Islets of Langherhans of the pancreas. Type 1 diabetes was formerly called type I diabetes, juvenile diabetes, juvenile onset diabetes, insulin-dependent diabetes mellitus and IDDM.

Type 1 diabetes is insulin dependent and usually develops in children, teenagers, or young adults under the age of 40. Without insulin, the patient produces ketone bodies as a by-product of fat metabolism, and type 1 diabetes might first be diagnosed when the patient develops ketoacidosis.

Some patients, particularly adults, retain enough residual beta cell function to prevent ketoacidosis for many years. However, people with this form of type 1 diabetes often eventually become dependent on insulin for survival.

Islet cell autoantibodies are markers of immune destruction and are present in most people with type 1 diabetes at the time when fasting diabetic hyperglycaemia is first detected. There is a genetic predisposition to autoimmune destruction of beta cells, and it is also related to environmental factors.

Type 1 diabetes is treated with insulin, diet and exercise.

■ Type 2 diabetes mellitus

Type 2 diabetes is the most common form of diabetes mellitus. People can develop it at any age, even during childhood, and this type of diabetes is becoming more frequently seen in young people. Type 2 diabetes was formerly called type II diabetes, adult onset diabetes, maturity-onset diabetes, non-insulin-dependent diabetes, and NIDDM.

Type 2 diabetes usually begins with insulin resistance. At first, the pancreas copes with the extra demand by producing more insulin. In time, however, the pancreas loses the ability to secrete enough insulin. Type 2 diabetes develops when the beta cells cannot produce enough insulin for the patient's needs, or because of insulin resistance.

This type of diabetes usually appears in people over the age of 40, although it often appears before then in South Asian and Afro-Caribbean people.

Type 2 diabetes implies a relative (rather than absolute) insulin deficiency. People with this type of diabetes do not usually need insulin treatment to survive and are sometimes undiagnosed for many years because their hyperglycaemia is often not severe enough to be symptomatic. However, they are at increased risk of developing macrovascular and microvascular complications, and type 2 diabetes should never be regarded as 'mild'.

Most patients with type 2 diabetes are overweight or obese, or have an increased percentage of body fat distributed predominantly in the abdominal region (Fig. 2.1).

Ketoacidosis is unusual in type 2 diabetes and, when it occurs, is usually associated with the stress of another illness or infection. Hyperosmolar non-ketotic coma (HONK) sometimes occurs in elderly patients and has a high mortality rate.

The risk of developing type 2 diabetes increases with age, obesity, and lack of physical activity (see Fig. 2.1). It occurs more frequently in women with a history of gestational diabetes (see below) and in patients with hypertension or dyslipidaemia. Its frequency varies in different racial and ethnic subgroups. It often runs in families: however, the genetics of type 2 diabetes are complicated and not fully understood.

Type 2 diabetes is managed with various combinations of insulin, oral hypoglycaemic agents, diet, and exercise. Patients with type 2 diabetes who are taking insulin should not be described as 'insulin dependent': they are 'insulin treated'.

■ Gestational diabetes

Gestational diabetes develops in some women who have hyper-glycaemia during the late stages of pregnancy. Although this form of

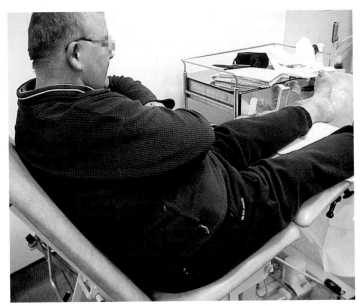

Fig. 2.1.   This patient with type 2 diabetes has a body mass index of 38. His diabetes is very poorly controlled and he also suffers from hypertension, hyperlipidaemia, and indolent neuropathic ulcers.

diabetes usually goes away after the birth, the mother has an increased risk of developing type 2 diabetes later.

AN EPIDEMIC OF DIABETES

At present, the world faces an 'epidemic' of type 2 diabetes. In the USA, Western Europe and developing countries, even quite young children are being diagnosed with type 2 diabetes. By the year 2020 it is anticipated that diabetic populations around the world will have doubled.

This is probably largely due to unsuitable diet, physical inactivity, and increased stresses associated with modern lifestyles, all superimposed on a genetic predisposition to diabetes in some people. However, the 'epidemic' might partly be the result of improved awareness of diabetes and better screening programmes.

GROUPS AT HIGH RISK OF DEVELOPING DIABETES

People at high risk of developing diabetes have the following characteristics:

- middle aged or older
- overweight or obese
- have a family history of one or more close relatives with diabetes
- are of African, Caribbean, or Asian ancestry
- have had gestational diabetes or have given birth to a baby weighing more than 9 lb
- have high blood pressure, low levels of HDL or high levels of triglycerides, and are physically inactive.

■ Patients with type 2 diabetes and the metabolic syndrome

This is a syndrome of hypertension, central obesity, and dyslipidaemia, with or without hyperglycaemia. Patients with metabolic syndrome are at high risk of developing macrovascular disease.

Often, patients with abnormal glucose tolerance or diabetes will have one or more other cardiovascular risk factors; this has been called syndrome X, the insulin resistance syndrome, or the metabolic syndrome, and is common in a wide variety of ethnic groups. It is possible that insulin resistance is the common aetiological factor for the individual components of the metabolic syndrome. Alone, each component of the syndrome conveys increased cardiovascular disease (CVD) risk, but in combination the effect is much more powerful. The management of patients with hyperglycaemia and other features of the metabolic syndrome aims to achieve good blood glucose control and also endeavours to reduce the other risk factors for CVD.

Features of the metabolic syndrome can be present for up to 10 years before detection of the glycaemic disorders. The metabolic syndrome with normal glucose tolerance identifies the subject as a member of a group at very high risk of future diabetes.

Aggressive early management of the metabolic syndrome can have a significant impact on the prevention of both diabetes and cardiovascular disease.

PREVENTION OF DIABETES

An American research study, the Diabetes Prevention Programme, has shown that people at high risk can reduce their chances of developing diabetes if they follow a low-fat, low-calorie diet, lose weight, and exercise regularly. The programme was effective for men and women, and worked particularly well for the 60+ age group.

Research into vaccines and gene therapy, as a means of preventing diabetes, is being undertaken.

DIAGNOSING DIABETES

One or more of the following tests may be used to diagnose diabetes:

- random capillary glucose test
- fasting plasma glucose test
- oral glucose tolerance test.

Random capillary glucose test

This is a one-off measurement of current levels of glucose in the blood. One single test result should not be used to diagnose diabetes: however, it is a very useful technique for close monitoring of glycaemic control. Many patients have their own small blood glucose meters and a supply of test strips for home blood glucose monitoring.

Fasting plasma glucose test

A fasting plasma glucose test is used to detect diabetes or prediabetes, and measures blood glucose after the patient has gone for a minimum of 8 hours without eating.

Oral glucose tolerance test

An oral glucose tolerance test can be used to diagnose diabetes or pre-diabetes. This measures the patient's blood glucose after at least 8 hours without eating and 2 hours after drinking a glucose-containing beverage.

MONITORING DIABETES

A useful test for monitoring glycaemic control is the measurement of glycosylated haemoglobin A1C (HbA1C). The average life of a red blood cell is 3 months and the level of glycosylation of haemoglobin is directly proportional to the amounts of glucose in the blood during the lifetime of the red cell. Thus the HbA1C measure is a useful guide to control over the previous 3 months.

At one time, poorly controlled diabetic patients who wished to please the healthcare professional and avoid admonishment would drastically reduce their glucose intake for 2 or 3 days before attending their appointment at the diabetic clinic so that their blood glucose measurement was low when tested at their clinic appointment. HbA1C testing means that patients can no longer fool healthcare professionals – or themselves.

SIGNS AND SYMPTOMS OF POORLY CONTROLLED DIABETES

The symptoms of undiagnosed or poorly managed diabetes include: fatigue, weight loss, insatiable thirst, polyuria, polydypsia, hunger, malaise, aches and pains, numbness and tingling, frequent skin infections and poor wound healing.

Some signs of uncontrolled diabetes are quite subtle, such as white, powdery patches on shoes or clothing (where glucose-laden urine has dried) or insects being attracted to spilled urine. One woman reported that the lavatory seat had become sticky where splashes of her husband's urine had dried on it.

Some patients with type 2 diabetes have such mild or absent symptoms that they are unaware that anything is wrong and may have had diabetes for many years before they are diagnosed, often as the result of investigations for another health problem or routine health checks. Sadly, diabetes is sometimes only diagnosed in such patients after they have developed a full house of complications. All patients not previously known to be diabetic but who present with foot ulceration, foot infection, or foot gangrene should be screened for diabetes.

THE HISTORY OF DIABETES MANAGEMENT

Methods of managing diabetes have changed greatly over the years. Up to the early twentieth century – before Banting, Best, Collip, and McLeod had developed insulin treatment – little could be done for patients with type 1 diabetes apart from offering a stay of execution.

■ The Allen diet

The Allen diet was developed to give type 1 patients a few months or years of living on 'borrowed time'. They were starved until their urine was glucose free and then only allowed enough food to maintain their urine in a glucose-free state. This approach offered them a slow lingering death from starvation instead of a quick death in ketosis.

Professor Michael Bliss, at the University of Toronto (where Banting and colleagues developed insulin treatment), has documented the discovery of insulin and the experiences of some of the first patients treated with insulin in the early 1920s in a fascinating book *The Discovery of Insulin* (3rd paperback edition, University of Toronto Press, Toronto, 2002).

■ The high-fat diet

Another early approach to diabetes management was the high-fat diet, in which carbohydrates were virtually eliminated from the diet and the patient was fed on fatty food.

■ After insulin …

After insulin treatment became available, diabetic diets were very rigid during the period from the 1920s to the 1960s. Dr Robin Lawrence at King's advocated strict portion control and issued patients with a little metal template for measuring precisely trimmed portions of bread. The modern approach to diet for people with diabetics is far more flexible.

MODERN TREATMENT OF DIABETES

With modern treatment, many people with diabetes now survive for many years and can lead an almost normal life (Fig. 2.2). The aims of modern treatment are:

- To achieve blood glucose and blood pressure levels that are as near to normal as possible.
- To maintain a healthy lifestyle.
- To achieve effective management of dyslipidaemia and smoking.
- To prevent long-term damage to the eyes (retinopathy), kidneys (nephropathy), nerves (neuropathy), and heart and major blood vessels (cardiovascular disease).

Fig. 2.2 The gold medal awarded by Diabetes UK to patients after 50 years of diabetes.

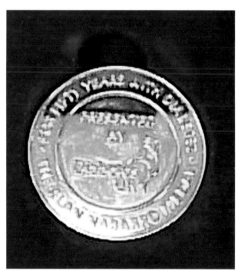

■ Diet and exercise

Diet and exercise are key components of modern diabetes management programmes. Patients need to understand that there are five groups of food and that a balanced diet will include components of each group.

The diet for people with diabetes is a balanced healthy diet – the same kind that is recommended for the rest of the population and which is low in fat, sugar and salt, with plenty of fruit and vegetables and meals based on starchy foods, such as bread, potatoes, cereals, pasta, and rice.

■ Modern management programmes
Dose adjustment for normal eating (DAFNE)

The new dose adjustment for normal eating (DAFNE) programme, first developed in Germany, helps type 1 patients to balance diet, exercise, and insulin intake in a much more flexible way and so lead a more normal life. The DAFNE programme is taught by diabetes specialist nurses and dieticians, and is available in a few centres in the United Kingdom.

DESMOND

DESMOND is a programme for type 2 patients with an emphasis on self-management and patients setting their own goals.

■ Common dietary pitfalls

These will vary with different populations. The author works in an area of South London with a large Afro-Caribbean population. Common dietary pitfalls among the foot clinic population include drinking too much orange juice (the announcement that this has 'no added sugar' does not mean that it is sugar free: in fact, orange juice is often used as a treatment for hypoglycaemia!); eating too much sweet fresh fruit, and especially the popularity of mangoes in season; and, of course, the 'hidden sugar' and high-fat content of processed foods, 'fast food', and some traditional foods. Podiatrists working in other areas will soon detect their own set of local problems.

Useful recipe books for people with diabetes are available from Diabetes UK (for address, see Appendix). However, 'normal' recipes are often suitable for people with diabetes or can be easily adjusted to reduce salt, unrefined carbohydrate and fat content.

Box 2.1 gives Diabetes UK's advice on eight steps to healthy eating for people with diabetes.

Box 2.1   **Diabetes UK's Eight Steps to Healthy Eating**

The following advice can be given to diabetic patients to help control blood glucose levels and blood fats as well as regulate weight:

Eat regular meals based on starchy carbohydrate foods such as bread, pasta, chapattis, potatoes, rice, and cereals. This will help you to control your blood glucose levels. Whenever possible, choose wholegrain varieties that are high in fibre, like wholemeal bread and wholemeal cereals to help maintain the health of your digestive system and prevent problems such as constipation.

Try and cut down on the fat you eat, particularly saturated (animal) fats, as this type of fat is linked to heart disease. Choose monounsaturated fats, e.g. olive oil and grapeseed oil. Eating less fat and fatty foods will also help you to lose weight. Use less butter, margarine, cheese and fatty meats. Choose low-fat dairy foods like skimmed milk and low-fat yoghurt. Grill, steam or oven bake instead of frying or cooking with oil or other fats.

Eat more fruit and vegetables – aim for at least five portions a day to provide you with vitamins and fibre as well as to help you balance your overall diet. A portion is a piece of fruit or a serving of a vegetable.

Cut down on sugar and sugary foods – this does not mean you need to eat a sugar-free diet. Sugar can be used as an ingredient in foods and in baking as part of a healthy diet. However, use sugar-free, low-sugar or diet squashes and fizzy drinks, as sugary drinks cause blood glucose levels to rise quickly.

Use less salt, because a high intake of salt can raise your blood pressure. Try flavouring food with herbs and spices instead of salt.

Drink alcohol in moderation only – that's two units of alcohol per day for a woman and three units per day for a man. For example, a small glass of wine or half a pint of beer is one unit. Never drink on an empty stomach, as alcohol can make hypoglycaemia (low blood glucose levels) more likely to occur.

If you are overweight, losing weight will help you control your diabetes and will also reduce your risk of heart disease, high blood pressure and stroke. Aim to lose weight slowly over time (1–2 lb per week) rather than crash dieting. Even if you don't manage to reach your ideal weight, losing a small amount and keeping it off will help with your blood glucose control and improve your overall health.

Don't be tempted by 'diabetic' foods or drinks. They are expensive, unnecessary, and have no added benefit for people with diabetes.

■ Exercise

People with diabetes are advised to undertake 30 minutes of brisk walking on at least five days a week. However, this advice might conflict with optimal management of foot problems. Patients with a history of foot ulceration might therefore need to take other forms of exercising, which are less likely to cause foot trouble, such as swimming or using an exercise bicycle.

Advice on weight loss for people with diabetes is available from Diabetes UK (Box 2.2).

Box 2.2   Diabetes UK's Ten Ways to Achieve Weight Loss

Set a realistic target weight. Do not get depressed if the weight comes off slowly. Losing any weight is better than losing none – or putting some on.

Aim to lose weight gradually. Losing 1–2 lb per week on average is good. By losing weight slowly but steadily, you can maintain satisfactory blood glucose control and the weight you lose is more likely to stay off. Avoid crash diets and 'slimming' products, which might look like an easy option. If you lose weight quickly you are more likely to regain the weight once you stop dieting.

Eat regularly. Don't skip meals! You will be more hungry, more likely to snack on high-calorie foods and more likely to eat extra food at your next meal. Missing meals will also make your blood glucose level more difficult to control.

Try to sit down and enjoy your meals. Eating more slowly helps your body to recognize that you have eaten properly.

Try to take up physical exercise. You do not need to be super-energetic and take up squash or aerobics. Gentle but regular exercise will help. Exercising with other people is less boring than exercising alone.

Weigh yourself just once a week at the same time of day in the same clothes. If you weigh yourself every day your weight will fluctuate and you might become disheartened at not seeing any improvement.

Choose high-fibre foods such as wholemeal bread, wholemeal chapattis, wholegrain cereals, wholewheat pasta, brown rice, fruit, and vegetables. These tend to be more filling than highly refined foods and although they seem strange at first one rapidly becomes accustomed to them.

Cut down on fat – use less butter or margarine and use easily spreading low fat alternatives:
- avoid adding extra fat or oil to foods
- grill, bake, microwave, or steam/poach food instead of frying it
- limit the amount of biscuits, cakes, pastries and crisps – even reduced fat ones – that you eat
- low-fat dairy products such as skimmed milk, cottage cheese and diet yoghurt are better for you than full-fat products.

Try to cut down on your alcohol intake:

- Alcohol contains a lot of calories and is an appetite stimulant.
- A pint of bitter contains about 190 calories.
- A pint of ordinary strength lager contains about 175 calories.
- Spirits contain about 55 calories per pub measure.
- White wine contains 113 calories per average glass.
- Diet drinks are virtually calorie free.
   Food is an important part of daily life. Continue to eat a variety of foods and to try new recipes.

■ Drugs for treating diabetes

Diet and exercise alone are often unable to control diabetes and in these circumstances it is necessary to resort to drugs (Fig. 2.3; for further details, see below). Drugs commonly used in diabetes include:

- insulin
- oral hypoglycaemic agents.

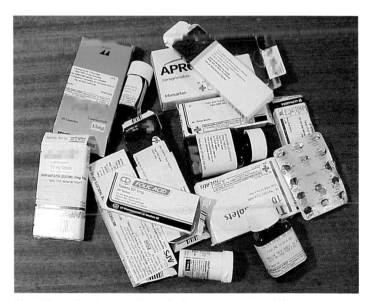

Fig. 2.3   Achieving good metabolic control can be difficult: one patient is on 14 different drugs.

Other treatments for diabetes include:

- pancreas transplantation
- islet cell transplantation
- folk remedies.

Pancreas transplantation
Pancreas transplantation is a complicated and risky procedure and is usually offered only as a combined renal pancreas procedure.

Islet cell transplantation
Islet cell transplantation is still in its infancy. Transplantation procedures involve long-term treatment with immunosuppressive drugs to prevent rejection.

Traditional folk remedies
Some of the substances used traditionally to treat diabetes, such as karela (bitter gourd) and 'bush tea' might exert a mild hypoglycaemic action but they should not be used except as part of a properly supervised diabetes programme.

THE MAJOR COMPLICATIONS OF DIABETES

Diabetic complications include:

- heart disease
- stroke
- kidney disease
- blindness
- nerve damage – sensory, motor and autonomic – with associated problems
- peripheral vascular disease
- increased susceptibility to infections.

Who will get complications?
It was long suspected that patients with poorly controlled diabetes with chronic hyperglycaemia, hypertension, and hyperlipidaemia would develop the complications of diabetes. The results of two large diabetes studies have confirmed this view. The key message from these two studies is that failure to control type 1 and type 2 diabetes greatly increases patients' chances of developing complications.

The Diabetes Control and Complications Trial (DCCT)

The Diabetes Control and Complications Trial was a large study following thousands of newly diagnosed type 1 patients in many different centres in the USA. There were two arms of the trial: one group of patients was offered normal advice and teaching and achieved average control; the other group achieved very tight control with special help, intensive education, and regular contact with and support from healthcare professionals, who offered them incentives to achieve good control. The study was stopped early when it was found, after several years, that the tight control group had significantly less microvascular disease. However, the tight control group had more episodes of hypoglycaemia.

The study was important because it confirmed that tight control of type 1 diabetes will delay or prevent the onset of complications. Sadly, many of the patients in DCCT in the tight control arm of the study were unable to maintain excellent blood glucose control long term but relapsed once they were released from the constraints of the study and no longer had access to super-special care and support. Achieving excellent control of type 1 diabetes is a lifelong battle and is easier said than done.

UKPDS

The other important study was UKPDS – the United Kingdom Prospective Diabetes Study – a large multicentre study of patients with type 2 diabetes in the United Kingdom. The late Professor Robert Turner from Oxford masterminded the study. UKPDS revealed that control of hyperglycaemia, hypertension, and hyperlipidaemia was an effective way of preventing or delaying complications in people with type 2 diabetes.

■ Screening patients for the presence of complications

The onset and development of complications may be insidious and symptom free, so patients need to be screened.

Investigations for the detection of diabetes complications
To detect metabolic problems

- Measurement of blood glucose to detect hyperglycaemia and hypoglycaemia.
- Measurement of HbA1C to monitor long-term control.
- Measurement of blood pressure to detect hypertension.

● Measurement of ketones to detect ketoacidosis.
● Tests to monitor renal function, including:
  ● microalbuminuria testing to detect the first signs of nephropathy
  ● measurement of protein in urine
  ● serum creatinine measurement (Box 2.3).

Eyes
The eyes need regular screening (at least annually). Screening may include:

● examination with ophthalmoscope
● retinal photography
● fluorescene angiography.

All of these tests help to detect the presence and extent of diabetic retinopathy.

The feet
Details of investigations for foot complications are given in Chapter 3.

Infections
Tests for the presence of infection include measurement of:

● body temperature
● C-reactive protein
● fibrinogen
● white blood cell count and numbers of particular cells.

These tests can help the clinician to assess the presence and severity of infection and the efficacy of treatments.

Box 2.3   Serum creatinine ranges

- Normal: serum creatinine of 80–120 μmol/L.
- Mildly impaired: serum creatinine of 120–200 μmol/L.
- Moderately impaired: serum creatinine of 200–400 μmol/L.
- Severely impaired: serum creatinine of > 400 μmol/L.
  Even mildly impaired renal function necessitates a review
of medication. Readers are referred to pages 118 and 119 of
A Practical Manual of Diabetic Foot Care (Blackwell Science, Oxford,
2004) for full details of antibiotic adjustments for renal patients.

Management of diabetes and its complications was greatly improved when home blood glucose monitoring became available. It is a quick and easy test.

Renal transplantation, renal dialysis, laser treatment for retinopathy, and coronary arterial bypass grafts are now widely available, and pancreas transplantation and islet-cell transplantation programmes are being developed.

■ Macrovascular disease

Macrovascular disease affects the:

- heart
- brain
- peripheral vessels.

The heart

The main diabetic cardiac complication, and a major cause of death, is myocardial infarction. Neuropathy affecting the heart can also lead to sudden death and arrhythmias, and cardiac symptoms might also be masked by neuropathy ('silent' myocardial infarction). There may be pain in the chest, arm, or jaw. Signs of cardiac failure include peripheral oedema and raised jugular venous pressure.

Cardiac problems in diabetes are managed with:

- drugs
- angioplasty
- bypass (coronary artery bypass graft – CABG).

The brain

Cerebrovascular accident – stroke – is a major cause of death among people with diabetes. Control of hypertension is essential for stroke prevention.

Peripheral vessels

Diseased peripheral vessels lead to the development of:

- ulcers
- gangrene
- amputations.

For treatments, see Chapter 6.

▩ Microvascular disease

Microvascular disease affects the:

● eyes
● kidneys
● nerves.

The eyes

Retinopathy is the most common ocular complication of diabetes, and includes:

● background retinopathy
● preproliferative retinopathy
● proliferative retinopathy.

Another common problem is development of cataract.

Abnormal growth of the retinal vessels can lead to intraocular bleeding, fibrin deposition, and retinal detachment. Untreated retinopathy is one of the most common causes of blindness in adults (Fig. 2.4).

For proliferative retinopathy, laser therapy is used to destroy or seal off new blood vessels, which are fragile and prone to bleeding. Pan retinal laser treatment reduces new vessel formation. It is important that patients realize that laser treatment will usually not improve vision, but that it can prevent deterioration.

Vitrectomy is undertaken after bleeding into the vitreous humour of the eye (from friable new vessels), which fails to resolve. This both affects the patient's vision and makes examination of the retina difficult. Vitrectomy involves surgical removal of vitreous humour and blood and replacing them with saline.

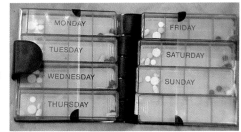

Fig. 2.4 A compartmentalized pillbox filled by the district nurse enables a blind patient who lives alone to take the right tablets at the right time.

When cataracts develop the lens of the eye becomes cloudy. Treatment involves removal of the lens and replacement with an artificial lens.

Iritis (uveitis)
Young type 1 diabetics with autonomic neuropathy may have a higher than usual amount of iritis, an acute inflammation of the eye, which presents with a red, painful eye that needs urgent medical treatment. There may be a further underlying systemic cause such as rheumatoid arthritis or ankylosing spondylitis. Iritis is usually treated with eye drops.

The kidneys (nephropathy)
Nephropathy is insidious in the early stages. Diabetic patients should be tested regularly for microalbuminurea, an investigation that can detect nephropathy at a very early stage. Patients with nephropathy should attend a joint renal/diabetes clinic.

Renal impairment means that special precautions must be taken before prescribing medication.

Treatments for nephropathy include:

● diet
● drugs (most importantly to control hypertension).

End-stage renal failure
Treatments for end stage renal failure include:

● continuous ambulatory peritoneal dialysis
● haemodialysis
● renal transplant.

The nerves – neuropathy (autonomic, sensory, and motor)
Autonomic neuropathy affects:

● blood pressure (postural hypotension)
● bladder (urine retention, urinary tract infections)
● gut (gastroparesis, diabetic diarrhoea)
● impotence (and arousal problems)
● heart.

▦ Postural hypotension

This complication of diabetic neuropathy can be quite incapacitating. When patients change posture – as from lying to sitting, or from sitting to standing – the blood pressure falls and the patients feel giddy and unsteady, might lose consciousness, and can suffer falls and injuries.

▦ Diabetic diarrhoea

This is caused by autonomic neuropathy of the gut, leading to episodes of uncontrollable diarrhoea, often nocturnal. Some patients are unaware that their diarrhoea is a diabetic complication. Before the diagnosis is made, it is necessary to exclude other causes.

Oral tetracycline often relieves symptoms.

▦ Impotence

Many men with diabetic neuropathy suffer from impotence. Some use penile implants, injections of papaverine into the corpus cavernosum of the penis, or drugs such as Viagra. Many men are embarrassed to mention their problem; they might become depressed and feel hopeless.

▦ Gastroparesis

This complication of neuropathy prevents the stomach from emptying: meals can remain in the stomach for many hours. Symptoms include weight loss and vomiting. This is a very serious complication and is treated by optimizing diabetic control, drugs (including domperidome and low-dose erythromycin to increase stomach motility), or surgery.

▦ Mononeuropathies

Acute femoral neuropathy

This presents with pain and muscle wasting on the front of the thigh. Abdominal neuropathy can mimic malignancy, presenting with pain and apparent swelling of one side of the abdomen. These get better after a few months.

Foot drop

The patient is unable to dorsiflex the foot and needs to be fitted with an ankle foot orthosis.

Nerves of diabetics are very sensitive to injury. Patients should be advised not to rest their arms on their elbows and to opt for elbow crutches rather than underarm crutches to avoid pressure damaging the nerves.

Pain

People with diabetes commonly complain of pain, which may be acute or chronic. A hyperglycaemic state can lower the pain threshold. Management of acute painful neuropathy is discussed in Chapter 7.

Chronic aches and pains are common. Pain in the diabetic foot should always be taken seriously.

Positive prayer sign

To detect this, the patient is asked to press his palms together as if praying. Sometimes he is unable to do this and a large gap between palms of the hands is evident. Many patients with this positive prayer sign have microvascular disease.

Hyperglycaemia

Hyperglycaemia is the state of increased amounts of glucose in the blood. It can occur as a result of lack of insulin, reduced levels of insulin, or insulin resistance. Hyperglycaemia is detected by measuring random capillary glucose from a small blood sample. However, a more useful test is haemoglobin A1C (HbA1C) measurement, which gives a good idea of average control over the previous 3 months (the life span of a red blood cell).

- The test measures glycosylation of red blood cells.
- Patients should be asked for their most recent HbA1C test result and encouraged to take an interest in it.
- An average HbA1C of <7% is associated with fewer long-term complications.

Hypoglycaemia

The state of hypoglycaemia, often called a 'hypo' by patients, occurs when blood glucose levels fall below 3.5 mmol/L. It is disagreeable for the patient.

- Symptoms include trembling, ravening hunger, sweating, and confusion.

● Patients who are persistently hyperglycaemic might have symptoms of hypoglycaemia with blood levels above the range that normally leads to hypoglycaemia.

Treatment of hypoglycaemia

Type 1 patients should carry their own supply of glucose but often do not, so a supply should always be available in the diabetic foot clinic. All the following contain 10 g of carbohydrate and are administered orally:

● 50 mL Lucozade®
● 100 mL natural unsweetened fruit juice
● 100 mL Coca Cola® or Pepsi® (not the diet version)
● 200 mL milk.

If patients are drowsy, unable to swallow or unconscious, the following can be used:

● Hypostop®: a glucose-laden gel that is rubbed over the gums.
● Glucagon: a hormone produced by the alpha cells of the pancreas, which causes the liver to break down deposits of glycogen, thus raising the blood sugar. It is delivered by intramuscular injection. Side effects include severe headache.
● Intravenous glucose: needed for unconscious patients with severe hypoglycaemia.

Hypoglycaemic unawareness

When the insulin-producing companies went over to the production of bioengineered human insulin in the 1980s, some patients reported that they developed reduced hypoglycaemic awareness and increased numbers of severe 'hypos' when they took human insulin. The reason for this was not clear at the time but is probably because control of diabetes was better on human insulin. With improved control came increased numbers of episodes of hypos. Episodes of hypoglycaemia reduce patients' awareness of hypoglycaemia and render them less likely to have warning symptoms of low blood glucose levels.

Some patients still insist on taking animal insulin because of their perception that human insulin causes hypoglycaemia, but supplies will become unreliable because many insulin manufacturers are discontinuing production of animal insulins.

All new diabetic patients in the UK should be started on human insulin.

▥ Ketoacidosis

The appearance of persistent ketones in blood or urine, in a patient with hyperglycaemia or high levels of glycosuria, indicates severe metabolic disturbance requiring urgent medical treatment. Patients should be advised to test for ketones when tests for glucose are repeatedly positive, and during periods of illness, particularly with infections. Reagent strips that are sensitive to ketones are available.

Patients on insulin should be warned not to stop taking insulin during periods of illness, even if they are not eating much: illness and infection greatly increase insulin requirements.

▥ Hypertension

Overly high blood pressure damages blood vessels and leads to macrovascular disease and kidney damage. Hypertension is detected with:

- blood pressure cuff – one off
- automatic BP cuff
- 24 hour BP monitoring.

Treatments include:

- drugs
- lifestyle changes.

▥ Hyperlipidaemia and triglyceridaemia

These are associated with macrovascular disease. Fatty deposits may be apparent on ear lobes or around eyes. They are diagnosed by blood test and treated with drugs (see below).

▥ Smoking

Tobacco use causes particularly severe health problems in diabetes. In addition to the common awareness that smoking can cause lung cancer, it is essential for people with diabetes to understand and believe that smoking damages blood vessels in the legs and feet, leading to peripheral vascular disease, ulcers, gangrene, and major amputations (Fig. 2.5).

Fig. 2.5   The foot of a heavy smoker who rolled his own cigarettes and underwent a major amputation soon after this photograph was taken.

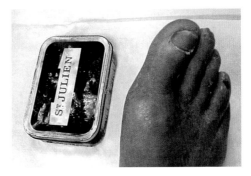

Tobacco is extremely addictive and healthcare professionals should not underestimate the effort it takes to give up smoking. Different approaches to smoking cessation include hypnosis and nicotine patches. Many NHS trusts have established special clinics for smokers, and diabetic patients who smoke should be strongly encouraged to enrol on a smoking cessation programme.

■ Obesity
The effects of obesity on the feet are numerous:

● Patients with a protruding abdomen will find it difficult to see or reach their feet, perform their own foot care, and detect problems early.
● In combination with neuropathy, obesity causes special problems because plantar pressures (associated with callus and ulcers) increase when the body mass becomes greater.
● It can be difficult for morbidly obese patients to walk and immobility can lead to pressure ulcers.

Control of the diabetes becomes more difficult with increasing obesity, and poorly controlled patients might be more susceptible to infection and poor wound healing.

Some obese people become socially isolated and rarely leave home, and it might be difficult to organize regular attendance for foot care.

Treatment of obesity

● Dieting, with simple dietetic advice, proper diets, weight-reduction groups.

- Psychotherapy.
- Exercising, either in a gym, or at home, is helpful, but may have deleterious effects on feet.
- Drugs.
- Surgery.

Surgical treatment of obesity

Where obesity is regarded as life threatening, patients are sometimes offered barosurgery, to reduce the working volume of the stomach. Two of the author's patients have undergone barosurgery and the results have been good, with considerable weight loss and improved control.

▓ Diets for diabetic complications

There is no evidence either way that diet plays a major part in promoting wound healing, but inadequate dietary intake is common in the elderly, frail and socially isolated. Dietary supplements such as zinc and vitamin B12 might be helpful.

Special renal diets for patients with nephropathy and chronic renal failure may slow down kidney damage. Limited quantities of high-quality proteins such as chicken, fish and lean meat, which produce fewer waste products, are included; added salt is precluded. High-potassium foods such as nuts and peanut butter are avoided, and fruit and vegetable intake is limited. Fluid is limited to six cups per day (including milk, soup, sauces, jelly and custard).

End-stage renal failure patients on dialysis need to maintain the balance of electrolytes, minerals, and fluid. Fluid restrictions are based on the amount of urine output and weight gain between dialysis sessions. Increased amounts of high-quality proteins are beneficial; high-potassium foods are avoided.

CONCURRENT MEDICAL CONDITIONS THAT MIGHT BE MORE COMMON IN PEOPLE WITH DIABETES

▓ Dermatological

- Diabetic dermopathy presents as harmless brown macular areas on the front of the shins, often following mild trauma.

● Bullosis diabeticorum: in this rare complication intraepidermal blisters develop with no history of trauma and heal without scarring: blisters may follow an episode of hypoglycaemia.
● Necrobiosis lipoidica diabeticorum: waxy atrophic lesions with telangiectatic centres develop, commonly on the front of the shins, which progress to ulceration in around one third of cases.
● Yellow nails.
● Haemosiderin deposition in neuropathic skin.

Orthopaedic

● Limited joint mobility.
● Fibrofatty padding depletion.
● Dupuytrens' contracture.
● Charcot's osteoarthropathy.
● Pathological fractures and slow-to-heal fractures.

Neurological

● Mononeuropathies, including:
 ● femoral neuropathy
 ● Bell's palsy.

Infections

Diabetic patients are particularly susceptible to many infections, including:

● Tuberculosis (TB)
● severe acute respiratory syndrome (SARS)
● boils
● carbuncles: like an enormous boil with several sinuses; sloughy, oedematous, cellulitic and painful. A very serious condition that needs urgent referral for antibiotics/surgery
● soft-tissue infections: cellulitis, septic vasculitis, necrotizing fasciitis
● osteomyelitis
● pseudomonal otitis externa: always refer-on patients with painful discharging ear immediately
● mucormycosis
● pneumonia
● Fournier's synergistic gangrene.

Diabetic patients with end-stage renal failure on continuous ambulatory peritoneal dialysis (CAPD) have an increased incidence of peritonitis.

DRUGS

It is difficult to manage foot patients properly unless details of their background and medical problems and treatments are known. All patients attending podiatrists should be asked to bring along details of their current treatment and medications.

■ Insulin

Human insulin is supplied in 100-unit containers and delivered in the following ways:

- subcutaneously
- intravenously
- by pump
- by infusion
- by sliding scale.

Sliding scale involves the use of short-acting insulin. The dose given depends on the level of blood glucose at the time of administration. Insulin is given at a dose determined by a preset algorithm. Sliding scale is used for acutely unwell, poorly controlled patients, and perioperatively, until things have settled down and the patient is recovering well.

Patients transferred to human insulin should be advised that the early warning symptoms of hypoglycaemia might be less pronounced than with animal insulin. Frequent hypoglycaemic episodes can reduce awareness of hypoglycaemia.

Dose adjustments of insulin may be required during:

- infection
- pregnancy
- periods of emotional distress
- in renal or hepatic impairment.

Occasionally, patients started on insulin develop acute pain (insulin neuritis).

Drug interactions with insulin

There may be interactions with:

- beta blockers
- monoamine oxidase inhibitors (MAOIs)
- corticosteroids
- diuretics
- oral contraceptives
- alcohol.

Types of insulin

- Lispro (Humalog®): prompt acting, given before meal.
- Lente Humulin R, Novolin R: short acting.
- NPH Humulin N, Novolin N: intermediate acting.
- Ultra lente (Humulin U®): long acting.
- Insulin glargine (Lantus®): long acting with no peaks.

Premixed combinations of regular and NPH insulins are available.

A company in India is now manufacturing and selling human insulin. Insulin companies selling in the United Kingdom include:

- Aventis
- Lilly
- Novo Nordisk.

Safe disposal of insulin needles is important. If patients are blind or not manually dextrous then special equipment is available to help them to self inject and maintain their independence.

Insulin pumps

These are used by a few patients. Advantages include:

- no need for daily injections
- steady release results in better control.

Disadvantages:

- indwelling needle
- if the pump malfunctions, patients can become ketoacidotic very quickly
- the needle might rub on clothes
- swimming and other sports can be problematic.

■ Oral hypoglycaemic agents

Box 2.4 gives the National Institute for Clinical Excellence (NICE) Guidelines for the use of oral hypoglycaemic agents. Oral hypoglycaemic agents include:

- sulphonylureas
- biguanides

Box 2.4 **NICE guidelines for the use of oral hypoglycaemic agents**

Information from NICE national clinical guidelines for type 2 diabetes – management of blood glucose:

- In people who are overweight (BMI >25) and whose blood glucose is inadequately controlled using lifestyle interventions alone, metformin should normally be used as the first-line glucose-lowering therapy.
- Metformin should be considered as an option for first-line or combination therapy for people who are not overweight.
- Insulin secretaqoques should be used in combination with metformin in overweight or obese people when glucose control becomes unsatisfactory.
- Insulin secretagogues should be considered as an option for first-line therapy when metformin is not tolerated or is contraindicated, or when people are not overweight.
- A generic sulphonylurea drug should normally be the insulin secretagogue of choice.
- Long-acting once-daily sulphonylureas may be useful where concordance with therapy is a suspected problem.
- Rapid-acting insulin secretagogues might have a role in attaining tight glucose control in patients with non-routine daily patterns.
- People should be offered a thiazolidinedione as oral combination therapy if they are unable to take metformin and insulin secretagogues as combination therapy, or if the HbA1C remains unsatisfactory despite adequate trial of metformin with insulin secretagogues.
- Acarbose can be considered as an alternative glucose-lowering therapy in people unable to use other oral drugs.

- thiazolidinediones
- prandial glucose regulators
- alpha glucosidase inhibitors.

Sulphonylureas: glibenclamide, gliclazide, glimepiride, glipizide, gliquizone

- Stimulate insulin secretion.
- May enhance action of insulin.

If type 2 patients become hypoglycaemic because of an overdose of sulphonylureas, they need admission to hospital because of the long-acting nature of these drugs.

Biguanides: metformin

- Augments glucose uptake in muscles.
- Reduces gluconeogenesis and intestinal glucose absorption.
- May induce lactic acidosis.

Thiazolidinediones: pioglitazone and rosiglitazone

- Enhance sensitivity to insulin in liver, adipose tissue and skeletal muscle.
- Increase uptake and storage of glucose.

They are used together with metformin or sulphonylurea. Patients should be monitored regularly for heart and liver problems.

Prandial glucose regulators: nateglinide and repaglinide

- Stimulate insulin release from beta cells of pancreas.
- They are taken just before each main meal.

Alpha glucosidase inhibitors: acarbose

- Retards glucose uptake from the intestines.
- Gastrointestinal side effects, with increase in gas formation from unabsorbed carbohydrate in the bowel.
- Patients taking combined sulphonylurea and acarbose should carry dextrose instead of sucrose because, in hypoglycaemia, sucrose absorption will be hindered by acarbose.

■ Antihypertensive agents
Diuretics
These include:

- loop diuretics (very strong)
- thiazide diuretics
- carbonic anhydrase inhibitors
- potassium-sparing diuretics (spironolactone, triamterene, amiloride).

Special precautions are needed when prescribing diuretics in diabetes and renal disease.

Hypolipidaemic agents

- Statins: these include atorvastatin, fluvastatin, pravastatin, and simvastatin.
- Fibrates: including benzafibrate, ciprofibrate, fenofibrate, and gemfibrozil.
- Omega-3 triglycerides: eicosapentaenoic acid (EPA).

An early case history

A patient of the author's was diagnosed with type 1 diabetes in 1923 (before insulin was widely available in the United Kingdom) at the age of seven. She was kept alive for 3 years on the Allen diet. She was so hungry that she ate the dog's biscuits, toothpaste, and flowers and leaves from the garden. She spent a short time in hospital on an alternative diet, where she was given nothing to eat but plates of fatty meat, swimming in grease, and begged her parents to take her home. After 3 years she was extremely emaciated, unable to walk, and on bed rest at home. Her life was saved by Dr RD Lawrence, a founder of the British Diabetic Association (now called Diabetes UK) who had diabetes himself. He admitted her to King's College Hospital and started her on insulin in 1926. At school in the 1920s and early 1930s, she was regarded as 'an invalid', excused games and made to attend part time only. However, after leaving school she led an active life, married and had a daughter, and recently died, aged 84, after 74 years on insulin.

Case history

A 63-year-old woman with type 1 diabetes of 47 years duration, proliferative retinopathy, and sensory and autonomic neuropathy, visited the foot clinic and mentioned that she had suddenly developed nocturnal diarrhoea, which came on without warning and was so severe that she was often unable to reach the lavatory in time. In one of her races for the bathroom she knocked her foot on the bedpost. She was not aware that her bowel problem could be due to diabetic neuropathy. Other causes of her problem were excluded. Although diabetic diarrhoea is not caused by infection, tetracycline frequently relieves the symptoms and this patient responded well to oral tetracycline.

- Bile acid sequestrants: cholestyramine, colestipol.
- Nicotinic acid derivatives: acipimox
- Antiplatelet agents: most diabetic patients should be on aspirin or clopidogrel.

MANAGEMENT OF END-STAGE RENAL FAILURE

■ Dialysis

Different types of dialysis are:

- continuous ambulatory peritoneal dialysis (CAPD)
- continuous arteriovenous haemofiltration (CAVH)
- continuous cycler assisted peritoneal dialysis (CCPD)
- nocturnal intermittent peritoneal dialysis (NIPD)
- haemodialysis.

The most commonly used techniques are CAPD and CAVH. For CAPD, a Tenchnikov catheter is inserted into the peritoneal cavity. Dialysis fluid can be inserted and drained-out several hours later through the catheter. Waste products diffuse across the peritoneum and are removed in the fluid. Fresh fluid is then inserted. CAPD is usually performed at the patient's own home. It is very expensive but cheaper than haemodialysis and the patient does not need to spend many hours at the dialysis centre. However, peritonitis is a common complication and many CAPD patients have very high creatinine levels.

Haemodialysis is usually performed within a renal unit, but some patients have a machine at home. It is a very expensive technique and every week the patient needs to spend two or three sessions, lasting several hours each, on a machine. Fluctuations of blood pressure can precipitate atheroma and vascular access can be a problem.

■ Renal transplantation

This is probably the gold standard treatment for diabetic patients in end-stage renal failure. However, transplanted patients are very vulnerable to infections and diabetic foot problems and need well-organized foot care (preferably within the renal unit to avoid the need for additional hospital appointments). These patients are on multiple drug regimens.

■ Drugs for diabetic renal patients
Erythropoietin

Erythropoietin is used to prevent anaemia, which is common in chronic and acute renal failure patients because their kidneys stop producing sufficient amounts of renin.

Immunosuppressants

These are used to prevent transplant rejection.

- Azathioprine is a cytotoxic drug that inhibits DNA synthesis. It prevents the proliferation of lymphocytes in response to the newly introduced antigens in transplant patients.
- Ciclosporin is more selective than azathioprine. It inhibits lymphocyte replication and the production of interleukin 2 (T cell growth factor). Neoral® is a formulation of ciclosporin; its absorption is less dependent on bile and so blood levels are more predictable.
- Tacrolimus is a macrolide lactone with potent immunosuppressant activity. It can be used first line or in patients refractory to ciclosporin and other immunosuppressant regimens. It inhibits the formation of cytotoxic lymphocytes as well as inhibiting lymphokine formation. It is not dependent on the presence of bile for absorption.

- Sirolimus inhibits lymphocyte activation, so allograft rejection is suppressed. It is used initially in combination with ciclosporin and corticosteroids, and then with just corticosteroids, to prevent organ rejection in renal transplantation.
- Mycophenolate prevents proliferation of T and B lymphocytes and also inhibits antibody formation and the generation of cytotoxic T cells. Used with ciclosporin and corticosteroids, it reduces the incidence of acute rejection in renal transplantation.
- Basiliximab is a monoclonal antibody which prevents binding of interleukin 2, the signal for T cell proliferation. It is used with Neoral® and corticosteroids to prevent rejection of renal transplants.
- Daclizumab also prevents binding of interleukin 2. The selective action reduces the immune response that causes acute rejection without affecting other immunocompetent cells.

All immunosuppressants reduce the ability of the body to fight infections and atypical infections, particularly fungal, may develop.

Immunosuppressant drugs include Cellcept® (Roche), Imuran® (Glaxo Wellcome), Neoral® (Novartis), Prograf® (Fujisawa), Rapamune® (Wyeth), Sandimmun® (Novartis), Simulect® (Novartis) and Zenapax® (Roche).

The renal unit should always be consulted when diabetic renal patients develop foot problems and changes to drug regimens are considered.

■ Renal tips!

- Patients on haemodialysis might be on heparin and will therefore bleed freely, so podiatrists should be wary when debriding the feet close to a dialysis session.

Case history

A 47-year-old man with type 2 diabetes, proliferative retinopathy treated by laser, nephropathy and obesity (body mass index 35) was determined to lose weight but had not succeeded with any weight-loss regimens and continued to gain weight. He then decided to try the popular Atkins diet, after consulting his GP and the renal physicians. After 3 months he had lost 15 kg, was able to reduce his insulin, and his plantar callosities greatly improved.

● If patients on CAPD or haemodialysis need antibiotics it is sometimes possible for these to be administered via a dialysis line or within dialysate fluid.

PREGNANCY

Diabetic patients who are planning to become pregnant should be referred to the diabetic clinic for preconception education and careful follow up. It is essential to optimize diabetic control before and during pregnancy.

METABOLIC CONTROL AND SYMPATHY FROM HEALTHCARE PROFESSIONALS

Podiatrists should try to be sympathetic to the problems that people with diabetes have in controlling their hyperglycaemia. Diabetes is a life sentence. Patients can never forget their diabetes, even for a day (Fig. 2.6). Constant vigilance is needed to optimize control, and

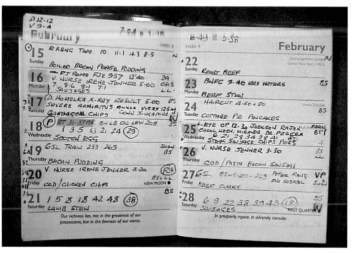

Fig. 2.6 A week in the life of a patient with foot ulcers. Podiatrists should be aware of how difficult life can be for their diabetic patients. People with diabetic foot ulceration can never take a holiday from their diabetes.

much of the joyous spontaneity of life is lost in the constant attempt to balance food intake against energy expenditure, current stress levels, and illness.

It is very easy to criticize patients for 'non-compliance' and podiatrists, while always supporting the need for good metabolic control, should be sympathetic to the problems their patients face as they try to live as normal a life as possible.

3 Examining the diabetic foot

A man whose blood
Is very snow broth; one who never feels
The wanton stings and motions of the sense.

William Shakespeare, Measure for Measure I. IV. 57

Looking at diabetic feet regularly, and acting rapidly on any problems found, is the key to success for patients and for healthcare practitioners. Diabetic feet should be checked at every visit to the diabetic clinic. It is important to make a careful examination and assessment of the feet before making any decisions about treatment or referrals. However, the podiatrist's (and the patient's) time is extremely valuable and it is important not to waste time with unnecessary procedures.

Two types of diabetic foot examination can be undertaken as follows:

- basic examination
- advanced examination.

All people with diabetes should undergo either a basic foot examination or an advanced foot examination at least once a year.

Basic screening of the diabetic foot does not have to be done by podiatrists but can also be performed by other healthcare professionals who have been carefully trained to assess the situation and react appropriately to the findings.

The basic foot examination should only take a few minutes. Its aims are to:

- detect the presence of significant problems
- ensure that the patient understands foot care and footwear
- refer the patient on if necessary.

The advanced foot examination has the following aims:

- to assess the current state of foot health in more detail

- to review the current treatment programme to ensure that it is optimal
- to act upon the findings.

THE BASIC EXAMINATION

This should detect:

- neuropathy
- ischaemia
- deformity
- swelling
- ulcer or other breaks in the skin
- infection
- gangrene
- previous major or minor amputation.

Both feet and lower limbs are visually inspected and palpated, not forgetting the interdigital regions, the area at the back of the heel and the nails.

Neuropathy

Neuropathy is detected by testing with a 10-g monofilament on the apex of the hallux and other pre-agreed sites.

Ischaemia

Ischaemia is detected by:

- palpating the pedal pulses
- checking the temperature and colour of the feet.

Deformity

Deformity is detected by inspecting and palpating the feet for:

- claw toes
- raised arch
- limited joint mobility
- bony prominences.

Oedema

The examiner inspects the feet and lower limbs for pitting oedema and compares the two feet to see if one is more swollen than the other.

▓ Callus

The skin is inspected for callus and corns. These may be associated with fissures, colour change or blistering under the callus (Fig. 3.1).

▓ Ulcers

The skin is inspected for breaks, including:

- blisters
- splits
- burns
- ulcers.

▓ Infection

The skin is inspected and palpated for:

- colour change
- increased warmth
- swelling
- discharge
- bad smell
- pain.

▓ Gangrene

Cold discoloured areas are detected by visual inspection and palpation. If none of the above is present, the patient is unlikely to get into serious trouble. However, the examiner should also check the shoes for:

Fig. 3.1 Heavy callus with speckles of blood within is an important warning sign of impending neuropathic ulceration.

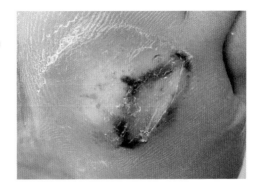

- size
- style
- state of wear
- suitability.

The examiner should gain an overall impression of whether the feet are being looked after well, and ensure that the patient is able to understand and undertake basic foot care.

▌ Action to be taken after the basic foot screen

If all is well, a further appointment for 1 year's time should be made.

If neuropathy or neuroischaemia, deformity, callus or swelling of the feet is detected, the patient needs an advanced assessment by a podiatrist.

If ulcer, infection or gangrene is detected the patient needs to be assessed urgently by a multidisciplinary diabetic foot team including a podiatrist.

Training of other healthcare professionals in how to conduct the basic foot screening can be imparted by podiatrists.

THE ADVANCED EXAMINATION

The advanced examination should ideally be performed by a podiatrist, who then decides by whom the patient should also be seen. (At King's Diabetic Foot Clinic, new patients are first assessed by podiatrists before being seen by the full multidisciplinary team.) The advanced examination for high-risk patients is in three sections:

- classification
- staging
- taking control.

▌ Classification

The advanced examination begins with a classification of the feet. The classification allocated depends on the detection of neuropathy or neuroischaemia. The foot with a combination of neuropathy and ischaemia is called the neuroischaemic foot.

It is rare to encounter a diabetic foot patient who has ischaemia and no neuropathy. The management of purely ischaemic feet is similar to the management of neuroischaemic feet except that pain is more of a problem and even gentle debridement may be painful.

Without knowing the class of the foot it is impossible for podiatrists to make suitable decisions as to:

- treatment
- referrals
- follow up.

Neuropathy

Four different types of neuropathy might be present in the diabetic foot:

- autonomic neuropathy
- motor neuropathy
- painful neuropathy
- sensory neuropathy.

The signs and symptoms of neuropathy are as follows:

Autonomic neuropathy

- dry skin
- fissuring
- distended dorsal veins (Fig. 3.2)
- warm foot
- increased blood flow
- bounding pulses.

It can be confirmed by autonomic function tests.

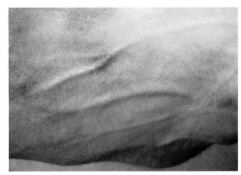

Fig. 3.2 Distended veins on the dorsum of the neuropathic foot are a sign of autonomic neuropathy and arteriovenous shunting.

Motor neuropathy

- Clawed toes
- Raised arch
- Foot drop
- Muscle wasting.

The podiatrist should test for weakness and resisted movement.

Painful neuropathy

Acute painful neuropathy presents as burning pain, usually in a stocking distribution, which is worse at night and may be associated with contact discomfort. Treatments are discussed in Chapter 7.

Sensory neuropathy

- Feelings of coldness
- Feelings of tightness
- Feeling as if walking on cotton-wool
- Numbness.

Simple tests for detecting sensory neuropathy include:

- 10-g monofilament
- Achilles tendon pinch
- Applying pressure to the nail plate.

More complex, quantitative tests for detecting sensory neuropathy are:

- biosthesiometer (but this instrument has been largely replaced by the neurothesiometer)
- neurothesiometer.

The podiatrist can quantitate the degree of sensory neuropathy present by using a 10-g monofilament. Another method uses the neurothesiometer, an instrument that delivers a vibratory stimulus to the foot; the stimulus increases in strength as voltage to the machine is increased.

Patients who cannot perceive the pressure from the 10-g monofilament, or a vibratory stimulus of 25 volts or above from the neurothesiometer, lack protective pain sensation and are at risk of ulceration.

Complications
Complications of the neuropathic foot include:

- nail problems
- dry skin
- painless callus
- dermal fissures
- plantar ulceration (Fig. 3.3)
- cellulitis and soft tissue infection
- osteomyelitis
- wet gangrene
- neuropathic oedema
- osteoporosis
- pathological fractures
- Charcot's osteoarthropathy.

Fig. 3.3   Plantar ulceration over the first metatarsal head of a neuropathic foot.

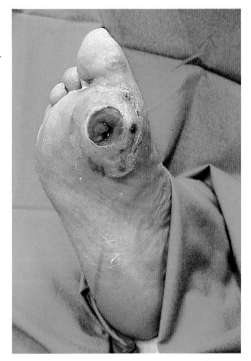

Ischaemia

Signs and symptoms of ischaemia include:

- absent pulses
- cold foot
- bright pink colour (sunset foot), pallor, or bluish discoloration
- atrophic skin and nails.

Ischaemia can be quantitated by means of a sphygmomanometer and hand-held Doppler. Even if the pulses are clearly present the podiatrist might still wish to measure the pressure index in order to have a baseline against which to measure any future deterioration.

Complications of the neuroischaemic foot include:

- intermittent claudication, which is often absent due to neuropathy and distal location of arterial disease
- rest pain, which might be reduced or absent depending on the degree of concurrent neuropathy
- marginated ulceration (Fig. 3.4)
- cellulitis or other soft tissue infection

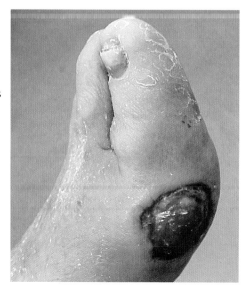

Fig 3.4 A large ischaemic ulcer on the medial border of a neuroischaemic foot. The patient has hallux valgus and wore unsuitable shoes which did not accommodate the deformity.

- wet gangrene (in the presence of infection)
- dry gangrene (avascular gangrene)
- acute ischaemia.

Classifying the foot in this way is not an arbitrary procedure. The care offered to the patient will differ according to whether the foot is deemed neuropathic or neuroischaemic in the following ways:

If the foot is neuropathic then:

- It is a 'forgiving' foot with an excellent capacity to heal.
- Sharp debridement is usually painless.
- Sharp debridement can be 'aggressive': making the foot bleed is not necessarily a bad thing.
- Callus is a common precursor of neuropathic ulceration.
- There is no need for further vascular assessment if at least one pulse in each foot is easily felt.
- Total contact casting is the gold standard treatment for indolent ulceration or acute Charcot's osteoarthropathy.
- Shoes for the neuropathic foot with plantar callus or ulcer should protect the sole of the foot and the dorsum of the toes: many patients need a shoe with a deep toe box, which can accommodate a cradled, total-contact insole.
- If failed healing or frequent relapse occurs there may be a role for the orthopaedic surgeon or podiatric surgeon in the management of the neuropathic foot.
- Neuropathic patients with good blood flow to the foot are at risk of Charcot's osteoarthropathy and their education should reflect this.
- With good management of the neuropathic foot, major amputation is very unlikely.
- With optimal control and early detection, neuropathic ulcers should heal within 6 weeks.

If the foot is neuroischaemic then:

- It is an unforgiving foot with a poor capacity to heal.
- Patients with peripheral vascular disease frequently have concurrent cardiac, renal and cerebrovascular disease.
- Debridement can be painful.
- Debridement should be extremely cautious and podiatrists should try not to make the foot bleed.
- Ischaemia should be quantitated by Doppler (or transcutaneous oxymetry, Duplex scan or angiography).

- The services of the vascular team may be needed.
- Antibiotics will be used more readily in the neuroischaemic foot.
- Local anaesthetics delivered by injection should not be used on the neuroischaemic foot.
- The neuroischaemic foot is not at risk of developing Charcot's osteoarthropathy.
- The total contact cast is contraindicated for the neuroischaemic foot: a suitable alternative casting technique is the Scotchcast boot.
- Shoes for the neuroischaemic foot should be sufficiently long, broad and deep with cushioned insoles.
- Even with optimal control, including vascular intervention where appropriate, healing will be far slower than in the neuropathic foot and outcomes are usually worse.

■ Staging

Having classified the high-risk foot as neuropathic or neuroischaemic it is then possible to stage the foot and use the staging to determine the necessary treatment, follow up and referrals.

There are several different staging systems that could be used. However, the Simple Staging System of Edmonds and Foster is recommended for podiatrists because it is

- based on the natural history of the diabetic foot
- very quick and easy to remember and apply
- validated: stage predicts outcome
- practical: it can be used as a framework for constructing management programmes and ensuring that existing treatments are adequate.

The Simple Staging System was designed and tested by a multidisciplinary diabetic foot team including podiatrists. It runs as follows:

- Stage 1 is the normal foot with no neuropathy and no ischaemia.
- Stage 2 is the high-risk foot where neuropathy or neuroischaemia is present.
- Stage 3 is the ulcerated foot where tissue breakdown (including cuts, splits, fissures, blisters, burns and/or ulcers) is present.
- Stage 4 is the infected foot (Fig. 3.5).
- Stage 5 is the gangrenous foot.
- Stage 6 is the unsalvageable foot where major amputation is inevitable.

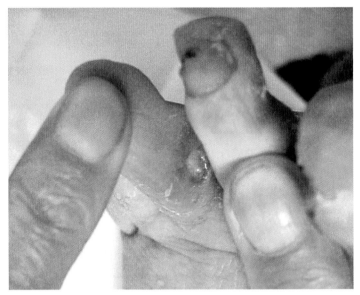

Fig. 3.5   An infected interdigital ulcer on a neuroischaemic foot.
The ulcer was not painful and the patient was unaware of its presence.

Once again, applying a stage to the diabetic foot is not an arbitrary decision. Once the foot has been correctly classified and staged it is then possible to use classification and staging as a framework for selecting a management programme for the patient.

There are six different aspects of management and taking control:

- mechanical control
- metabolic control
- microbiological control
- vascular control
- wound control
- educational control.

The final section of the advanced examination looks into which of the above aspects of control are needed for the individual patient. As patients move up the stages, control becomes more complicated and a greater number of aspects of control need to be taken into account.

- For Stage 1 patients (at low risk) the main emphasis will be on metabolic control and educational control.
- Stage 2 patients are at high risk and may need mechanical control and vascular control in addition to metabolic and educational control. Some stage 2 patients have Charcot's osteoarthropathy (for diagnosis and management see Chapter 7).
- Stages 3 and above need all of the six aspects of control to be examined.

Each of the above aspects of taking control is allocated a special chapter in this book.

Assessment of mechanical control

Assessment of mechanical control is needed for all patients at Stage 2 and above (see also Chapter 4) and will include:

- Examination of feet and shoes.
- Questioning patients about the range of footwear or offloading devices used.
- Searching for signs on the feet (red marks, callosities, blisters, ulcers) of abnormal mechanical forces that might be due to wearing unsuitable shoes or not wearing shoes.
- Assessing the shoes to ensure that they are appropriate and suitable, looking at the wear marks on the soles and checking the shoes both inside and out.
- Deciding what method of offloading is most appropriate short term and long term and discussing problems with the multidisciplinary team.
- Liaising, where necessary, with the orthotist regarding manufacture, issue and upkeep of footwear and orthotics.
- Persuading patients to follow offloading advice.

Assessment of metabolic control

This is needed for all patients (see Chapter 2). Podiatrists should know:

- if there has been a recent check of HbA1C, blood pressure, lipids, and the results of these tests
- the smoking history
- if the patient is being seen regularly by the general practitioner or the diabetic clinic

- whether the eyes are checked regularly and the ocular status
- whether the blood pressure is checked regularly
- whether the body mass index is elevated or the patient is obese
- the renal status
- current problems with the diabetes control.

The patient might need further education or referral to the physician or diabetes specialist nurse.

Assessment of educational control

This is needed for all patients (see Chapter 9). The podiatrist should explore whether patients:

- know how to look after their feet and are capable of delivering foot care
- perceive themselves to be at risk
- understand what foot care is needed and why
- know what is suitable footwear
- remember the danger signs of actual or impending foot problems
- know what to do and where to go if problems develop or deteriorate.

Patients in higher stages will require further assessment relating to education geared to their specific stage, such as ulcer care, signs that ulceration and infections are deteriorating, methods of keeping gangrene dry, and early reporting of problems.

Assessment of microbiological control

This is needed for patients in Stages 3, 4, and 5 (see Chapter 5). The podiatrist should examine wounds and compare the two feet, searching for signs and symptoms of infection including:

- increased size, depth, undermining or sinus
- colour change to the wound bed or around the ulcer (Fig. 3.6)
- increased discharge
- increased odour
- pus
- swelling
- pain
- fever
- rigors
- malaise.

Fig. 3.6 This ischaemic ulcer, on the remaining foot of a major amputee, stopped healing and was reassessed. The wound bed is very pale, indicating poor perfusion, and there is cellulitis affecting the skin around the ulcer. The pressure index of the foot was 0.4 and no vascular intervention was deemed feasible. A wound swab grew *Staphylococcus aureus*. The patient was treated with oral flucloxacillin and the ulcer improved.

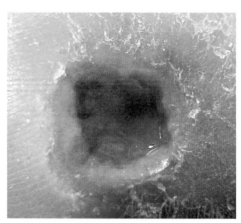

If any of these is found:

● swabs or tissue samples are taken and sent for microscopy and culture
● previous microbiology results and results of other recent investigations are checked
● further necessary investigations are undertaken.

If the foot is infected, decisions need to be taken regarding:

● antibiotic treatment
● whether hospital admission is necessary
● whether surgery is necessary.

Other members of the team will need to be consulted if the diabetic foot is infected.

Assessment of vascular control

This is needed for patients in Stages 2, 3, 4, and 5 (see Chapter 6). The following questions need to be asked:

● Is the foot ischaemic?

- If so, how ischaemic is the foot and what investigations (pulses, Doppler, $TcPO_2$, Duplex, angiography) will help to confirm the degree of ischaemia?
- Is the ischaemia critical?
- What treatments might be necessary (Fig. 3.7)?
- Can the patient wait to be seen in the vascular outpatient clinic or should the vascular team be asked to see him urgently?

Assessment of wound control

This is needed for patients in Stages 3, 4, and 5 (see Chapter 8). Is the wound:

- Adequately and sufficiently frequently debrided?
- Dressed with a suitable dressing appropriately fastened?

The following questions should also be asked:

- Who is dressing the wound?
- Is the wound regularly inspected?
- Is the wound improving or deteriorating?

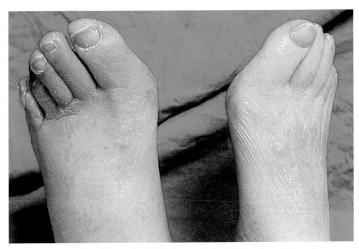

Fig. 3.7   A cold, pink, painful, ischaemic foot. The fourth toe is infected and the apex of the toe is blue and pregangrenous. The foot is critically ischaemic and needs urgent vascular intervention.

- Are any investigations needed (microbiology, X-ray, etc.)?
- How should the wound be treated short term and long term?
- Is referral necessary? To whom?
- Where should the patient be followed up and when?

In the beginning the practitioner might need to refer to a checklist to ensure that no aspect of taking control is unexplored. Podiatrists should trust their 'sixth sense', which, as they become more experienced, will tell them when all is not well or when further referral or investigation is needed. It is safest always to assume a worst case scenario. It is better to refer ten patients with non-malignant lesions to the dermatologists than to miss one malignant melanoma.

Taking action and referral pathways

The podiatrist should always ask:

- Whether the problem found lies within her area of expertise.
- Whether she can treat the foot by herself or whether she needs help, and if so, from whom.

When seeking help, podiatrists should beware of referring to the inexperienced! It is essential for podiatrists to be aware of the local situation, to get to know other practitioners in the field of diabetic foot care and to know where experienced and sympathetic help can be obtained. Unfortunately, some healthcare professionals have little interest in diabetic foot care. For this reason, it might sometimes be necessary to bypass a certain general practitioner and refer the patient directly to the accident and emergency department of the local hospital, or to ask for the patient to be seen by a particular physician or nurse in the diabetic clinic.

The following points are important:

- When the foot has a serious problem, the podiatrist should always telephone the people to whom the patient is to be referred to explain the situation and record that this has been done in the notes.
- Patients should also always be given a letter explaining the problem (a copy of which should be posted to the person who has been asked to see the patient). A copy should also be sent to the general practitioner and a copy retained in the podiatry notes.
- The patient should be asked to inform the podiatrist if any immediate problems arise with obtaining further treatment.

PATIENT INFORMATION

Podiatrists need to be well informed about their patients. The following information about high-risk diabetic foot patients needs to be gathered and recorded in the notes:

- age of the patient
- sex of the patient
- type of diabetes
- duration of the diabetes
- contact details of patient and next of kin
- name and contact details of general practitioner?
- name and contact details of whoever referred the patient to the podiatrist.

■ Complications and risk factors

- What diabetic complications, if any, are present?
- Does the patient have risk factors for the development of foot problems: neuropathy, ischaemia, deformity, swelling, callus, or any non-diabetic foot problems?
- Current medication
- Allergies
- Does the patient have any of the following current foot problems: ulcer, infection, gangrene, painful neuropathy, acute ischaemia, severe chronic ischaemia, fracture, and Charcot's osteoarthropathy? What is the duration?
- If so, how, where and by whom have they been treated?
- Does the patient have any previous history of foot problems? How, where and by whom were they treated? What was the outcome?
- Does the patient have other relevant health problems? If so, how, where and by whom are they treated?
- Is the patient's footwear adequate? If not, what is wrong with it and has the patient been advised?
- Has the patient been fully and correctly educated?

■ Future management

- What investigations are needed?
- What treatments are needed?
- Does the patient need referral onwards? To whom?

● Does the patient know what to do and where to go if new foot problems arise, or current problems deteriorate?

It is not necessary, when writing up the notes and examination findings, for the podiatrist to write a long essay. Notes recording the examination should be clear and succinct and written in black ink. They are a legal record and should stand up to scrutiny by others.

4 Offloading the diabetic foot

T'is not enough to help the feeble up,
But to support him after.

William Shakespeare, Timon of Athens I. I. 108

Offloading is a key area of managing the diabetic foot both in terms of preventing ulcers and healing ulcers. Throughout the world, offloading is an area where podiatrists and other healthcare practitioners often fail to achieve optimal care. It has often been said that it matters little what you put upon a foot ulcer in terms of dressings and topical applications so long as you take the pressure off. Foot ulcers are very rare in people with protective pain sensation because they are forced by pain to limp and rest, and thus offload the foot.

Offloading is necessary to prevent and heal ulcers because of the response of the diabetic foot to increased pressure, friction and shear. All of these forces can lead to inflammation, excessive callus formation, tissue damage and ulceration. If ulcers are not offloaded well then healing is impaired, the wound becomes chronic, infection can spread more easily, and amputation can result (Fig. 4.1).

Like dieters who are 'in denial' about how much they are eating, many diabetic neuropaths seem to be 'in denial' about how much they are walking. The aims of offloading are to reduce any abnormal and destructive mechanical forces to which the foot is subjected and thus to:

● achieve healing of ulcers and wounds
● prevent callus, ulcer or further injury.

When an ulcer is present, any pressure, frictional, or shearing forces applied to the wound should be regarded as abnormal and undesirable. It might therefore be said that when a foot wound is present the only acceptable level of offloading is total offloading. However, achieving total offloading is usually not feasible as there will be other conflicting aims such as:

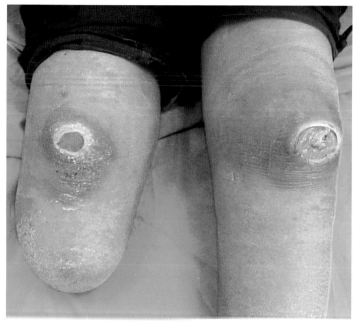

Fig. 4.1 This patient, who underwent major amputation for an infected neuropathic foot, was unable to wear a prosthesis because of fluctuating oedema, crawled around the house on his knees, which were also neuropathic, and developed ulcers.

- enabling the patient to get up and walk in a reasonable way
- achieving an acceptable level of activity
- helping the patient to achieve a reasonable quality of life.

Problems with offloading include:

- transferring excessive forces to adjoining or other parts of the foot or leg, which may cause new areas of callus or ulcers
- stiffness of joints
- muscle atrophy
- osteoporosis (a particular problem with extended periods of bedrest and in plaster casts).

HISTORICAL BACKGROUND OF OFFLOADING THE DIABETIC FOOT

Podiatrists and orthotists have traditionally been the members of the multidisciplinary team most involved in offloading, although some nurses (notably Sister Rosemary Clarke from the plaster room at Leicester Royal Infirmary) and surgeons (the late Paul Brand and Frank Tovey) have pioneered offloading techniques for diabetic patients. Dr RD Lawrence said that an ulcerated foot should not be put to the ground and that patients should use padded crutches for offloading.

Paul Brand, a great pioneer of offloading, who died in 2003, confronted the problem of leprosy patients with neuropathic ulceration or Charcot's osteoarthropathy and who were unable to take time off work. Brand, working in southern India, borrowed a technique previously used by a Dr DeSilva who used close-fitting plaster casts with minimal padding to achieve healing while the patients kept on their feet and continued to walk and work.

Sister Rosemary Clarke, who worked in the plaster room at Leicester Royal Infirmary, collaborated with Dr Felix Burden to develop the Scotchcast boot (see below).

Frank Tovey was a British surgeon who worked in India and developed the Tovey insole, a cradled insole that conformed precisely to the contours of the sole of the patient's foot. On his return to the UK he worked closely with Orthotist Mick Moss at Lord Mayor Trelaur Centre in Basingstoke. A Tovey-style insole is built on a last made from a plaster cast of the foot. The insole, with layers made of different densities of plastazote, incorporates a cradle to grasp the foot by the margins, thus reducing friction. The contours of the insole conform to the entire sole of the foot (including the medial longitudinal arch), which thus becomes a weight-bearing area. Because the forces are distributed over a larger area, any discrete sites of particularly high pressure are reduced because the total load-bearing area of the foot has been increased and individual areas are subjected to less pressure. Major problems with the original Tovey insole are that it occupies so much space that it frequently needs to be accommodated in a bespoke shoe, and the plastazote tends to bottom out after a few weeks.

In the early days of the Diabetic Foot Clinic at King's, patients with indolent neuropathic ulcers were offered bespoke shoes containing Tovey-type insoles. Significantly fewer patients relapsed in the group who wore their specially provided shoes than in a matched group of patients who refused hospital shoes and insisted on wearing their own shoes. Luigi Uccioli in Italy and Ernst Chantelau in Germany have also published studies demonstrating the efficacy of special footwear.

Many people with diabetic foot problems do not want to wear shoes that stigmatize them as being patients. Neil Baker, lead podiatrist in the Diabetic Foot Clinic at Ipswich, explored the problem of patients who do not use footwear provided by the hospital and found that many patients were not wearing prescribed shoes.

PRESSURE

Pressure can cause damage to the diabetic foot in three different ways:

- One episode of high pressure may cause direct trauma to tissues.
- Intermittent pressure may cause inflammation, excessive callus formation and cumulative tissue damage.
- Continuous pressure, even at a low level, may prevent circulation of blood to affected tissues, which then undergo ischaemic damage.

Common examples of damaging pressure

- *Pressure from tight shoes*: before patients have neuropathy they are accustomed to feeling their shoes on their feet. As neuropathy develops, when they try on shoes they might choose a pair which is too tight because it gives them the familiar sensation of feeling the shoes on their feet. If these new shoes are too tight they cause continuous pressure on the margins of the feet. Tight shoes also constrict the toes, preventing normal toe function and overloading the metatarsal heads.
- *Unrelieved pressure from lying in bed without moving*: this is a common event when frail diabetic neuropathic and neuroischaemic patients are admitted to hospital, not turned regularly, and not given pressure-relieving mattresses or foam wedges to offload their heels.
- *Pressure on the margins of the feet when oedema develops and the shoes become too tight*: this is a particular problem in the neuroischaemic foot, because patients with peripheral vascular disease often also have cardiac or renal problems causing peripheral

oedema. Swelling from infection or acute Charcot's osteoarthropathy can also result in pressure from a shoe that normally fits well but has become too tight because the foot is swollen.

● *Raised plantar pressures in neuropathic feet*: where a high medial longitudinal arch and claw toes lead to a reduced weight-bearing sole area.

● *Increased plantar forefoot pressures caused by fibrofatty depletion*: reduction of fibrofatty padding on the sole of the foot, which may be displaced forward by abnormally high plantar pressures or destroyed by ulceration or infection, reduces the foot's capacity to absorb pressure without damage to underlying tissues.

● *Localized areas of pressure caused by limited joint mobility*: examples include hallux rigidus, leading to overloading of the plantar phalangeal area at the toe-off phase of the gait cycle, (Fig. 4.2) and plantar flexion of the foot, due to limitation of dorsiflexion at the ankle, leading to increased plantar pressures on the forefoot.

● *Increased pressure from stiffening of the soft tissues*: this renders them less resilient.

Some diabetic feet may be more susceptible to damage from external mechanical forces than is normally the case, and the damage may be immediate, because the ability of the tissues to absorb tensile stress of the flesh is reduced (as in the case of 'tissue paper thin' skin in the elderly). Damage may also develop because of an abnormal response to injury (which may be due to neuropathy, ischaemia or renal problems) where a tiny defect becomes a large ulcer.

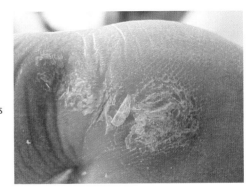

Fig. 4.2 Hallux rigidus leading to heavy callus under the great hallux and over the first metatarsal head. Without urgent debridement of callus this site will ulcerate. A rocker sole applied to the patient's shoe will help to offload the foot.

■ Other specific effects

Specific effects of diabetes and its complications on the foot, which may make patients particularly prone to damage from pressure, include:

- Weak bones, which are common in the neuropathic foot, possibly because of increased blood flow demineralising the bones, and may develop fractures, dislocations or Charcot's osteoarthropathy.
- Poor proprioception leading to abnormal mechanical forces being exerted on bones, joints and soft tissues.
- Unsteadiness from postural hypotension leading to falls and resulting injuries.
- Neuropathy, leading to lack of pain and unawareness of excessive pressure.

The need to reduce abnormally high mechanical forces on vulnerable sites is paramount. This can sometimes be achieved by:

- Diverting them to another area more able to cope with them.
- Spreading them out to eliminate foci of high pressure.
- Eliminating them: however, the only way to achieve this is either by total rest and elevation of the foot, which is rarely practical or accepted by the patient, or by using elaborate, expensive and cumbersome orthotics, such as the patellar tendon-bearing weight-relieving orthosis or the knee–ankle–foot orthosis.

In both the neuropathic foot and the neuroischaemic foot, the damage caused by excessive mechanical forces may not be easily perceived by the patient because of poor eyesight, lack of pain, and inability to reach the feet.

Oedematous or deformed feet are also very prone to mechanical damage, and renal feet are probably the most easily damaged of all.

Whatever stage the foot has reached, it can usually be offloaded effectively with a combination of podiatry, orthotics, and – occasionally – surgery. However, outcomes are more likely to be good if potential problems are detected early and acted on quickly.

Offloading is both a science and an art, and can sometimes only be achieved by trial and error; close supervision and follow-up of patients and offloading devices will be necessary. It is best if the orthotist works within the diabetic foot clinic so that support is available from the podiatrist and other members of the team. Multidisciplinary case conferences are essential for difficult cases.

Shoes and orthotics should be checked every day by the patient and at every clinic visit by the podiatrist.

A POSTCODE LOTTERY

At present, diabetic foot patients in the United Kingdom face a postcode lottery – large areas of the country have no adequate diabetic orthotics service, overstretched podiatry services and podiatric surgeons with no established role.

At large podiatric meetings, during audience discussions, one of the most frequent complaints is that good shoes and orthotics are not widely available for the high-risk diabetic foot. Even when an effective orthotics service is available, waiting lists may be long.

BIOMECHANICS

It is not within the scope of this chapter to explore the field of biomechanics in great depth. Biomechanics is a large and complex area: quantitation of problems and interventions, difficulties of precise measuring and repeatability and concordance between different practitioners ('a few degrees of posting' can vary wildly depending on who is assessing the patient) can all lead to problems in this area. To gain practical insights into biomechanics and the diabetic foot, readers are referred to the work of Dr Peter Cavanagh, who worked for many years at the Center for Locomotor Studies at Pennsylvania State University, USA, and has produced a very useful bibliography on the foot in diabetes. It was Peter Cavanagh who said that a diabetic foot patient should never be allowed to leave the clinic wearing the same pair of shoes that caused an ulcer.

Podiatrists who specialize in biomechanics must take great care when planning offloading interventions for the high-risk diabetic foot. In theory, Charcot's osteoarthropathy can be triggered by too aggressive an intervention, resulting in a rapid, unstaged change in the application of forces to the foot. Rigid orthotics can cause damage and should be used with great caution in the high-risk foot.

■ Common biomechanical abnormalities

Common sites of diabetic foot ulceration associated with specific biomechanical abnormalities are described below. The biomechanical abnormalities lead to development of 'pressure points' (areas of high pressure, friction or shearing stress), which are sites for callus formation, blistering or ulceration.

■ Sites of ulceration

The most common ulcer sites are:

- The toes: on the dorsum associated with claw or hammer toe deformity; on the apex associated with claw toe, on the nail bed, associated with onychogryphosis or onychauxis, or on the plantar surface, associated with hallux rigidus (see Fig. 4.2) or other toes affected by limited joint mobility.
- The plantar surface of the neuropathic foot, where the ulcer may be associated with fibrofatty padding depletion, the presence of a bony prominence, plantar scarring from previous ulceration or surgery, and plantar flexion deformity, all of which can lead to overloading.
- The borders of the ischaemic foot, which may be subjected to pressure from tight shoes and need to be offloaded in extra depth, wide-fitting shoes. Pressure needs to be reduced if ulceration is to be prevented or healed.

ACCOMMODATING THE DIABETIC FOOT

The aim is to alleviate problems including:

- Congenital or acquired deformities, which are accommodated in suitable footwear that might need to be tailor made.
- Oedematous feet and ischaemic feet, which are accommodated in shoes with adjustable fastenings. These can adapt to fluctuating volume and are sufficiently long, broad and deep to avoid pressures on the margins of the foot.
- Limited joint mobility and biomechanical abnormalities, which are compensated for by means of surgery or orthotics or shoes.
- Calluses on pressure points, which need to be regularly debrided and offloaded.
- Ulcers, which need debriding and offloading.
- Acute Charcot's osteoarthropathy, where feet need immobilization and offloading.

The majority of diabetic foot ulcers are on the toes. In the neuropathic foot the sole is vulnerable, in the neuroischaemic foot the borders are vulnerable. Sites of ulceration in the neuropathic foot and the neuroischaemic foot are tabulated in Tables 4.1 and 4.2.

MANAGEMENT OF MECHANICAL CONTROL

Offloading problems can be prevented or improved with callus debridement and provision of suitable footwear or orthotics.

■ Callus removal

Full details of techniques for safe removal of callus are found in Chapters 6 and 8. Sharp debridement is the treatment of choice: keratolytic agents should always be avoided in the high-risk diabetic foot.

Table 4.1 *Common sites of ulceration in the neuropathic foot, causes and solutions*

Site	Cause	Solution
Over dorsum of toes	Claw or hammer toe	Deep toe box
Over apices of toes	Claw or mallet toe	Felt or silicone rubber toe prop, apical pad, surgery
Interdigitally	Tight shoes, prominent interphalangeal joints	Broad toe box
Plantar toes and pp1	Hallux rigidus or limited joint mobility in lesser toes	Rocker sole
Metatarsal heads	Lack of fibrofatty padding, plantar flexion deformity, high arch	Cushioned cover pad
Rocker bottom	Charcot foot	Cradled insole
Medial prominence	Charcot foot	Felt sock, bespoke shoe
Medial or lateral malleolus	Charcot ankle	Bespoke shoe or boot, CROW

CROW, Charcot restraint orthotic walker.

Table 4.2 *Common sites of ulceration in the neuroischaemic foot, causes and solutions*

Site	Cause	Solution
Medial border and lateral border	Pressure from shoes, oedema	Wide-fitting shoes
Around the borders of the heel	Loose shoes, fissures	Snug-fitting heel cup, emollient for dry skin, debridement of fissures
Apices of toes	Short shoes	Appropriate shoe length
Beneath thickened toe nails	Trauma to nails or fungal infection	Regular reduction of nails and deep toe box

■ Neurovascular corns and calluses

It is important to ensure that callus is removed as evenly as possible, otherwise subsequent uneven pressure on the skin may lead to the development of a neurovascular corn or callus. These lesions, where nerves and small blood vessels have invaded callus tissue, are painful and difficult to treat, and are uncommon in people who have never attempted to pare their own corns and calluses.

■ Benefits of callus removal

Plantar callus removal can:

● reduce plantar pressures
● prevent ulceration.

In addition, debridement of callus from around neuropathic ulcers can:

● prevent extension
● promote healing (see Chapter 8).

However, in addition to removing callus regularly (and always before it develops speckles of blood and enters the pre-ulcerative state) it is essential to offload the area of high pressure that led to the callus formation. The key way to achieve this is by means of footwear.

▥ Suitable footwear

Types of footwear available to diabetic patients include:

- high street
- mail order
- off-the-shelf stock shoes
- modular shoes (these are stock shoes that can incorporate certain fixed modifications; podiatrists sometimes carry out other shoe modifications such as inserting balloon patches)
- bespoke shoes, which are sometimes used in association with orthotic devices.

▥ Acceptability of footwear

Many diabetic foot patients find it difficult to accept weight-relieving treatments (see Chapter 10) because of the resulting constraints on social or working life or for reasons of aesthetic acceptability and fashion consciousness. Well-functioning footwear is important but if the footwear does not appeal to the patient or fit in with his lifestyle, it is likely to end up in the back of the wardrobe. On the one hand, it is essential to produce footwear that is acceptable to the patient. On the other hand, when endeavouring to accommodate severely deformed diabetic feet, the podiatrist and orthotist can only go so far in conceding to the demands of the patient regarding size and style of the shoes. However, issuing shoes that the patient will not wear is useless, and sometimes it might be necessary to achieve a compromise and issue shoes that are suboptimal but are better than the shoes the patient has previously been wearing.

For reasons of cost to the diabetic foot service, acceptability and convenience, patients should be accommodated in high-street or off-the-shelf shoes whenever possible. This should be achievable in all Stage 1 and many Stage 2 diabetic feet. Sports shoes and boots are excellent for everyday wear.

OTHER WEIGHT-RELIEVING TECHNIQUES

▥ Insoles

Insoles can be made by podiatrists, orthotists (Fig. 4.3) or technicians. They may be simple (flat bed, usually one layer, provided in stock shoes) or compound (moulded, usually made of two or three

Fig. 4.3 The orthotist is a key member of the multidisciplinary team. He is fitting a poron sink to an insole.

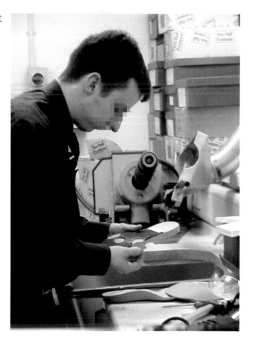

layers of different densities and may contain sinks or extra padding to offload specific areas).

Problems with insoles include:

- bottoming out
- inaccurate fit
- insufficient cushioning
- overly space occupying.

Insole materials include:

- silicone
- vitrathene (great care should be taken when prescribing rigid insoles or rigid orthotics for the diabetic foot)
- plastazote
- poron
- ethyl vinyl acetate (EVA).

▨ Injections to augment fibrofatty padding

Lack of or displacement of fibrofatty padding is a common cause of callus formation and ulceration. Interventions to address this problem include a technique pioneered by Dr Saul Balkin, an American podiatrist, who has for many years advocated the use of injections of liquid silicone to:

● augment fibrofatty fading
● cushion bony prominences
● prevent the development of corns, calluses and ulcers.

However, this technique is not widely used by others. This is partly due to early problems with migration of silicone (overcome by using many injections of smaller quantities of silicone) and fear of potential hazards of systemic effects of silicone, which were exacerbated by problems with silicone breast implants and mass litigation. Patients are also often reluctant to undergo multiple injections.

In the 1980s studies were also performed with collagen, widely used for cosmetic treatment to plump out wrinkles in the face. For treating diabetic feet, collagen was rendered more durable by incorporating extra disulphide bridges. The collagen was injected to augment fibrofatty padding at sites of callus formation and previous ulceration. However, the technique, although minimally invasive and promising, was expensive, and never used in diabetic foot patients in the United Kingdom except in research studies.

▨ Silicone rubber

This is a very useful substance for modelling bespoke orthotics to cushion and protect bony prominences, to prevent the development of interdigital corns and ulcers, and to improve the function of claw toes.

▨ Silicone gel

This comes in transparent sheets, which can be cut to size and used to cushion bony prominences and sites subjected to pressure, friction and shearing forces. It is also available already incorporated into toe sleeves, socks, and other appliances or as stick-on pads. It is excellent at reducing mechanical forces.

▨ Vitrathene

This rigid thermoplastic material is not widely used for high-risk diabetic patients.

▨ Plastazote

This lightweight material was formerly widely used but has a tendency to 'bottom out' and has largely been replaced by EVA (ethyl vinyl acetate).

▨ EVA

This corky (in colour and consistency) material has similar mechanical properties to plastazote but is less liable to 'bottom out'. It is widely used in modern insoles for people with high-risk diabetic feet.

▨ Poron

This provides extra cushioning to compensate for lack of fibrofatty padding, cushion bony prominences and reduce areas of high pressure.

▨ Felt padding

Felt padding is made of felted sheep's wool backed by hypoallergenic adhesive so that it can be stuck onto the foot to deflect pressure and correct function. Edges of felt pads should be bevelled. Types of pads include:

- dorsal cavity pads for toes
- horseshoe pads to deflect pressure from prominent dorsal interphalangeal joints
- toe props
- apical U'd pads to deflect pressure off the apex of a toe
- plantar cover pads
- U'd plantar cover pads (Fig. 4.4)
- metatarsal pads to improve function
- U'd pads around bony prominences
- felt to cover bony prominences such as the tibial crest, tuberosity of navicular, styloid process and medial and lateral malleolus within a total contact cast
- felt tongue pads can be fitted to shoes when the girth has stretched. This ensures that when the laces are tightened the foot is gripped firmly to eliminate friction.

▨ Dangers of appliances made of adhesive felt directly applied to the foot

Use of adhesive felt is not entirely without problems. Trouble can be caused by:

- allergy to adhesive
- injury to skin when padding is pulled off

Fig. 4.4 Traditional adhesive semicompressed felt is a good short-term method of reducing pressure. This patient will wear a 'U'd' plantar cover pad until his new insole is ready. He will check around and under the pad at frequent intervals to detect any problems early.

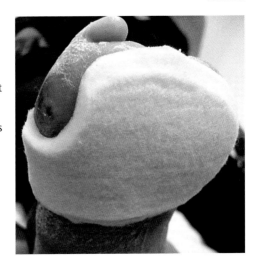

- rendering the shoes too tight.
- masking of ulceration or infection.

One very serious case was seen by the author in the early 1980s at King's where infection and gangrene had developed beneath a felt pad.

Case study

A 7 mm semi-compressed felt plantar cover pad was applied to the foot of an 84-year-old diabetic woman after debridement of a corn, and left in place for 3 weeks. The patient had profound neuropathy, lived alone, was frail, and followed instructions – not to remove the pad before the community domiciliary chiropodist called again – to the letter. After 2 weeks the foot was painful but the patient did not remove the pad because of the instructions she had been given. When the pad was removed, deep ulceration, severe infection, and extensive gangrene were found. She underwent surgical debridement of the first ray of her left foot, which took nearly 9 months to heal.

Because of the difficulties of early detection of infection under opaque dressings or pads, felt padding should ideally be applied only to the diabetic foot as a temporary measure while attempts are made to solve the offloading problem with alternative methods such as shoes, insoles, or orthotics. Pads should be lifted regularly for foot inspection and removed immediately if there is any discomfort or pain in the foot, the diabetes is unstable or the patient develops fever or feels unwell with 'flu like symptoms.

Special precautions with felt padding

- Ensure patient has no allergy to the adhesive.
- Ensure pads are carefully removed to avoid tearing skin.
- Do not apply padding to atrophic, ischaemic feet.
- Check the foot regularly, lifting the pad to inspect underlying skin.

■ Walking aids

Walking sticks

These must be sturdy and specially fitted with a non-slip rubber on the end. Some patients are reluctant to use a stick because of the perceived association with old age and ill health. Sticks are very useful for unsteady patients as a balance aid but do not really provide adequate offloading for an ulcerated foot.

Crutches

These should be of the modern 'elbow' type. Old fashioned crutches, which take weight under the arms, can cause severe nerve palsies in diabetic patients, whose nerves are particularly susceptible to compression injuries. Crutches are used when it is essential to entirely, largely or partially eliminate weight bearing from the foot or lower limb, or to support an unsteady patient.

The use of crutches is physically demanding. Patients need to be fit, not liable to falls, and able to maintain balance when the eyes are closed.

All patients who are issued with crutches should be trained in their use by a suitably qualified healthcare professional and, in particular, taught to go up and down stairs. Their length should be carefully adjusted for the individual patient. Unsteady patients risk falls. Weak and frail patients, and the severely visually impaired, are unsuitable for crutches.

Zimmer frames and similar devices

These lightweight walking frames are widely used. Again, there is a perceived stigma because these devices are associated with old age and ill health. (When the author was in hospital with Guillain–Barré syndrome in 1983 she well remembers both how useful her Zimmer frame was, and how unhappy and stigmatized she felt at being obliged to use it!) Zimmers are extremely useful for patients who are very unsteady, elderly, or frail. There are frames with wheels at the front, which can be pushed forward as well as lifted. Zimmers can be fitted with drink holders and hooks for handbags. Any competent handyman can fit a shelf with a cushion to a Zimmer, on which the patient can rest the knee to ensure offloading of an ulcerated foot, although this is not available commercially.

Some elderly patients use shopping trolleys around the house to carry things they need and as a walking aid to provide extra stability.

Wheelchairs

These may be pushable or self-propelled by the patient, and are essential for patients who require entire offloading or are unable to cope with walking even when assisted by crutches or Zimmer. It is possible to fit a plank extension under the seat cushion on which the patient can elevate the foot and leg. Some very sophisticated versions of the wheelchair are available. These aids can be very expensive. Lightweight, collapsible, folding wheelchairs are useful. Extra cushioning is needed if a plank extension is used. Obese patients may need bespoke wheelchairs, which can take many weeks to make, and the result may be a delayed hospital discharge.

Adaptations including cushioned extensions to elevate a leg and clip on baskets, trays, shelves, or drinks carriers are available.

Wheelchairs are not suitable for all patients. It can be dangerous for blind or severely visually impaired patients to self-propel a wheel chair. Many patients are extremely reluctant to use a wheelchair. Wheelchairs are frequently borrowed without permission, stolen or lost, and should be guarded carefully, especially within hospitals.

It might be necessary to modify a patient's house or flat for wheel chair use (fitting ramps, widening door spaces, fitting stair lift) and these modifications can be very expensive.

Electric cart or buggy

Several of the author's patients have purchased these. They are extremely useful, enabling the patient to get out and about without having to walk or transfer. They run on rechargeable electric batteries and have a distance capacity of several miles.

Four-wheel drive vehicles, snowmobiles, jet skis, etc.

Imagination is necessary if patients with limited walking capacity do not become housebound and socially isolated. Small four-wheel drive vehicles are available, enabling patients to go off the road in quite rough country. These are very useful for patients who live in the countryside, become depressed at being 'stuck at home', and who particularly miss aspects of country life such as taking walks or exercising the dogs. Patients can participate in family holidays and expeditions when suitable aids are available.

Case study

A 65-year old man, who was not known to be diabetic, developed a sore on the sole of his foot. It was not painful and he applied a sticking plaster. Four weeks later, when it had not healed, he visited his general practitioner who performed a random capillary glucose measurement, and type 2 diabetes was diagnosed. He had bounding pulses and a neuropathic ulcer was diagnosed and treated in the hospital diabetic foot clinic.

The patient lived on his own, in a ground-floor flat, and went out every day, shopping and visiting friends. The ulcer failed to heal despite provision of bespoke shoes and insoles. He was reluctant to accept a total contact cast or use a wheelchair. However, he agreed to purchase an electric cart. The small model he obtained had a range of 10 miles, with a rechargeable battery, and he used it for all his outside activities, including visits to the hospital. Within 4 weeks of purchasing the cart, his ulcer healed and has not recurred.

CASTS

Casting is the mainstay of diabetic foot ulcer management. Types of cast include:

- total contact cast
- Scotchcast boot
- Aircast and other removable walking braces.

Total contact cast

The total contact cast (Fig. 4.5) is widely regarded as the gold standard (best and most effective) treatment for indolent neuropathic ulcers and acute Charcot's osteoarthropathy. This may be because the total contact cast enforces compliance, because the patient is unable to remove it. The total contact cast was first developed for agricultural labourers in the developing world who had leprosy and neuropathic ulcers but who were unable to rest because they had to bring money home for their families. It is a close-fitting cast, made of plaster of Paris or, in the affluent West, of fibreglass casting tape. Bony prominences (tibial crest and medial and lateral malleoli) are padded with felt. A study by David Armstrong, an American podiatrist, and colleagues demonstrated better healing of neuropathic ulcers in total contact casts than in Aircast products and special shoes.

Patients attending the total contact casting clinic should wear shorts or wide trousers to enable them to change their clothes while wearing a cast.

Fig. 4.5 The total contact cast is gold standard treatment for indolent neuropathic ulcer and acute Charcot's osteoarthropathy. It is not suitable for neuroischaemic feet.

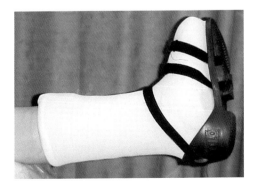

The materials needed for each total contact cast are as follows:

- A foam pyramid to elevate the leg so that it is not in contact with the leg rest. A roll of towels can be used if this is not available.
- Stockinette (a length double the distance from the tips of the toes to the knee. The size of stockinette used will depend on the diameter of the patient's leg).
- 5-mm adhesive felt: two circles with a diameter of 5 cm, which cover the malleoli, and a strip 3 cm wide and long enough to reach from the tibial crest to the ankle. If there are additional bony prominences more pieces of felt will be needed to protect them.
- Cast padding: usually three rolls, 7 cm wide, per cast.
- Casting tape: usually three rolls, 7 cm wide, per cast but if the patient is very heavy more rolls will be needed. Wet casting tape should not come into contact with podiatry chairs, clothes, trolley tops or bare skin. Podiatrists performing casting should always wear gloves.
- A pair of gloves for each operator (special casting gloves incorporating silicone are ideal). Wet casting tape should not be touched with the bare skin: it can cause severe dermatitis and patients should be warned.
- Plastic sheeting to protect the podiatry chair.
- A bucket of warm water in which to dip the casting tape.
- Written advice for the patient.
- A vibrating cast saw for adaptation or removal of cast.

All the materials for each individual cast should be laid out in advance on a trolley top in the order in which they will be applied. This helps to avoid inadvertent omissions.

The casting procedure

Total contact casting is a job for two podiatrists: one holds the foot in a plantigrade position, supports the leg and assists in rubbing the tape to a smooth finish. The other selects and applies the materials. The stages of the procedure are as follows:

1. A layer of stockinette is applied to the foot and lower leg. Enough stockinette is included to provide a lining for the cast and also to cover the hard, rough surface of the completed cast to prevent trauma to the contralateral leg. The extra material,

which will be used to cover the cast, is gathered up over the knee during the casting procedure and then rolled down to cover the completed cast.

2. Small pieces of cast padding are applied between the toes to reduce pressure and to absorb perspiration.

3. The foot is held in a plantigrade position and the stockinette adjusted to fit over the end of the toes, trimmed and taped. Any creases in the stockinette around the ankle are cut out and taped flat.

4. The felt strip is applied to the tibial crest and the circles of felt are stuck over the malleoli. If the tuberosity of the navicular or the styloid process are prominent then pieces of felt should be stuck over them, and any other bony prominences.

5. The area to be covered with cast padding stretches from the tibial tuberosity to the tips of the toes. At the proximal end, three layers are applied and the operator then works down the leg, overlapping the padding by one-third each time it goes round the leg. The distal area, around the toes, needs extra padding, and layers of padding should be fanned over the ends of the toes and back so that they are well protected by at least three layers of padding.

6. The casting tape is removed from its foil packaging. This should be done only when the operators are ready to use it, because it hardens quickly on contact with air. The roll of tape is dipped into the bucket of warm water and submerged until bubbles stop rising. It is then lifted out and gently squeezed to remove excess water. Speed of hardening of the tape will increase proportionally to the heat of the water used; therefore experienced operators may want to use hot water, and beginners start with cold water.

7. The tape is applied. It covers a smaller area than the padding material because a 2.5 cm strip of padding at the top of the cast is left clear of tape. The tape application begins with three layers at the proximal end of the cast, applied 2.5 cm below the proximal end of the cast padding (the tape edge should be well clear of the tibial tuberosity). The operator then works distally moving down the leg and overlapping the tape by one-third each time it goes round the leg. When the toe area is reached the tape is fanned over the ends of the toes and back to construct a strong protective toe box. During the entire procedure it is essential for

the plantigrade position of the foot to be maintained: the job of the person who is holding the foot is to maintain a good position at all costs.

8. When all the tape has been applied it is rubbed gently so that the layers of tape adhere to each other. Both hands of the main operator and one hand of the person holding the foot in position may do this. At all times the casting tape is handled with the flat of the hands avoiding pressure from finger tips which might cause dents and subsequent ulceration. At this stage, some practitioners like to apply gentle pressure to flatten the area of the cast covering the sole, for improved stability when the patient is standing and walking.

9. The excess layer of stockinette is rolled down from the knee to cover the cast. The hard proximal edge of the cast is thus snugly enclosed in cast padding and stockinette on both sides. Any excess material at the distal end is trimmed and taped. The stockinette adheres closely to the tape and makes a neat finish. If any adaptations are to be made (see bivalved cast and windowed wound protection cast below) this should be done before Stage 9.

10. The patient is allowed to hang the leg down, being careful that no part of the cast is pressing against a solid object that might dent it

11. After 30 min the operator performs a final check of the cast for strength and fit. The cast is gently pulled distally and pushed proximally to ensure that no pistoning movement of the cast against the leg is possible. If all is well, then the patient is allowed to walk.

Indications for use of the total contact cast are indolent neuropathic ulcer and acute Charcot's osteoarthropathy.

Patients with infection or ischaemia and patients who cannot be relied upon to attend regularly and follow advice should never be put into a total contact cast.

The patient's general practitioner and diabetes clinic should be informed that it is intended to apply a cast.

Potential problems include pressure points, rubs and breaks in the skin and infections, which may spread unperceived under the cast.

Courses for podiatrists to learn the technique of total contact cast manufacture are available at the diabetic foot clinic at King's College Hospital NHS Trust.

Adaptations to the total contact cast include the:

- removable bivalved cast
- windowed wound protection cast.

■ Bivalved cast

The total contact cast can be rendered removable after Stage 8 above. The cast is allowed to harden and then the front is cut out, the rough edges are bound with Elastoplast® tape, incorporating the layers of cast padding, and the two sections can be fitted together onto the leg and held in place with a crepe bandage. However, there may be excessive motion leading to iatrogenic lesions but the advantages are that the cast may be removed for wound inspection. (An illustration of the bivalved cast is shown in Fig. 7.8A, on p 207.)

The bivalved cast is used for patients with neuropathic ulceration or acute Charcot's osteoarthropathy where regular inspection of the leg is felt to be essential, or when patients live too far from the centre to attend quickly if problems arise. It may also be suitable for patients with previous history of severe and rapidly ascending infection; patients whose managing physician does not support the use of an unremovable cast, and patients with 'cast phobia'.

■ Windowed wound protection cast

This is a total contact cast but after Stage 8 the cast is allowed to harden and a removable window is then cut in the cast over the ulcerated area. At the edges of the window the underlying padding and stockinette are pulled through and drawn back over the rough edges of the window and taped in place. The edges of the window are thus padded to prevent injury. The piece of scotch cast which was cut out to create the window can have a centimetre of material removed from around the edges. The remaining piece of fibreglass can be covered with Profore® #1 (previously called Sofban®) padding and Elastoplast® to create a snugly fitting window which can be regularly removed for wound inspection and redressing of the ulcer. If it becomes mucky with exudate from the ulcer the padding can be removed and replaced with fresh padding and Elastoplast.

■ Scotchcast boot

The Scotchcast boot (Fig. 4.6) is a bespoke temporary boot made from an inner lining of felt and an outer shell made of fibreglass

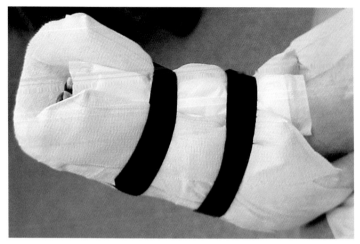

Fig. 4.6 The Scotchcast boot is an excellent treatment for neuroischaemic feet with marginated ulcers or gangrene.

casting material. It is useful for offloading the vulnerable margins of an ulcerated ischaemic foot, and also reduces pressures on the plantar surface of a neuropathic foot (although not so effectively as the total contact cast). Courses for podiatrists to learn the technique of Scotchcast boot manufacture are available at the Blackburn diabetes centre and at King's College Hospital NHS Trust. The materials needed for making each Scotchcast boot are as follows:

- A piece of stockinette long enough to cover the area from mid calf of the patient to 10 cm distal to the tips of the toes.
- A piece of 7-mm felt that is 5 cm longer than the maximum length of the foot and 5 cm wider than the maximum width of the foot.
- Two rolls of 5 cm cast padding.
- Three rolls of 5-cm casting tape (this must not be opened until it is needed: it hardens on contact with air). Wet tape must not come into contact with the skin of the patient or the bare hands of the operator, and will damage the surface of trolleys and patient chairs.
- One roll of 5-cm Elastoplast® tape.

● A pair of casting gloves.
● A bucket of warm water.

A cast saw is not needed because all the casting tape is cut with scissors while still soft.

The manufacturing procedure is as follows:

1. The piece of stockinette is applied to cover the area from mid-calf to 10 mm beyond the tips of the toes.
2. The piece of felt is applied to the sole of the foot with the non-adhesive side in contact with the skin. The felt extends from the tips of the toes to 5 cm up the back of the heel and up each side of the foot for 2.5 cm (triangles are cut out of the felt so that the fit around the heel is snug).
3. Cast padding is wrapped very loosely around the foot and ankle to hold the felt in place and provide a thick layer of padding. If the padding is applied too tightly it will cause difficulties later: it should be just tight enough to keep the felt in place.
4. The packet of cast tape is now opened. Three lengths are cut from it. Each piece should be as long as the sole of the foot. These are overlapped to create a piece of fibreglass that will cover the sole of the foot.
5. The remaining casting tape is dipped into the warm water until the bubbles stop rising and then, after shaking off excess water, it is wrapped around the foot, keeping well within the area covered by padding.
6. Excess fibreglass is trimmed away around the entire border of the foot, ensuring that it does not extend onto the malleoli, up the back of the heel, or above the felt on the sides of the foot. All sharp corners of fibreglass are rounded off. The fibreglass covering the dorsum of the foot is lifted away, ensuring that as much of the underlying padding as possible is left behind.
7. The stockinette is folded back over the foot from each end.
8. The boot is wrapped in Elastoplast® tape.
9. While the fibreglass tape is still soft, the sole of the boot can be gently pressed against the floor to flatten it for subsequent ease of walking.
10. A felt 'tongue' is made to fill the gap left by removal of fibreglass material on the dorsum and thus protect the foot from any rubbing.
11. A removable cast sandal is issued.

At this stage the boot is an unremovable device. To make it removable, additional stages are needed as follows:

12. The dorsal area of the boot is cut open through the layers of Elastoplast®, cast padding and stockinette. *Note*: if the padding has been applied too tightly the boot will spring open and not retain its close fitting shape which is why previous instructions were given to wrap padding loosely around the foot.
13. The raw edges of the cut are sealed with Elastoplast®.
14. Ready-made straps of velcro are applied over the midfoot and high on the foot. These are adjustable to accommodate oedema and hold the boot and the felt tongue in place.

Scotchcast boots are useful for ischaemic patients with ulceration when footwear is not offloading the foot sufficiently and the patient is unwilling or unable to refrain from walking sufficiently to heal the ulcer. It is useful for patients with ischaemic gangrene. The Scotchcast boot is sometimes used for neuropathic patients with plantar ulceration or Charcot's osteoarthropathy, though the total contact cast is preferable.

■ Aircast walking brace

This is a below-knee bivalved walking brace lined by four inflatable air pockets. These can be blown up with a small hand pump to ensure a snug fit. The pump on the 'diabetic' version gives a pressure measurement to avoid over inflation. It looks rather like a ski boot. The footballer David Beckham wore one when he fractured a metatarsal shortly before the World Cup, since when a number of young patients have been very keen to wear an Aircast!

The Aircast brace improves the immediate offloading capacity of a foot clinic. It can be used for patients with indolent neuropathic ulceration or acute Charcot's osteoarthropathy but who are unsuitable for a total contact cast; the author has not used it for patients with ischaemia.

The Aircast walking brace cannot accommodate severe deformity but the plastic shell can be adapted with a heat gun to accommodate minor deformity.

■ The 'instant total contact cast'

Some practitioners have recently advocated use of a removable walking brace that has been wrapped in fibreglass tape so that the patient is no longer able to take it off. This enforces compliance and is quicker and cheaper than manufacturing the full total contact cast. However, many patients with indolent neuropathic ulceration or Charcot feet have such a degree of deformity that they need a bespoke cast, like the total contact cast.

▓ Problems associated with casts

Elderly or unsteady patients risk falls, and back problems may be exacerbated by leg length discrepancy.

OTHER OFFLOADING DEVICES FOR THE DIABETIC FOOT

Other useful offloading devices include the:

- Pressure-relieving ankle–foot orthosis (PRAFO)
- ankle–foot orthosis (AFO)
- patellar–tendon-bearing weight-relieving orthosis (PTB)
- Charcot restraint orthotic walker (CROW)
- knee scooter.

▓ Pressure-relieving ankle–foot orthosis (PRAFO)

The PRAFO (Fig. 4.7) is a removable, fleece-lined brace with a metal frame that offloads the heel area very effectively. The PRAFO can be worn in bed to prevent or offload bedsores on the heel of the neuropathic or neuroischaemic foot, and can be walked in for short distances.

▓ Ankle–foot orthosis (AFO)

This plastic splint is moulded to the back of the calf and foot to support the foot and ankle and prevent excessive mobility. It is used to treat Charcot feet and ankles in the recovery phase and to stabilize cases of excessively mobile ankle and foot drop.

▓ Patellar–tendon-bearing weight-relieving orthosis (PTB)

This is something of a last resort, when offloading of foot and ankle is essential and the patient has to walk. The device is very cumbersome and heavy, rather like a below-knee amputation (BKA) prosthesis.

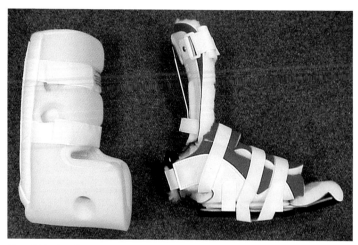

Fig. 4.7 Heel protection is essential for bedbound, high-risk patients. The pink foam device and the pressure-relieving ankle–foot orthosis (PRAFO) are both useful. They maintain the foot in a plantigrade position, preventing foot drop. In the PRAFO a patient can walk a little.

■ Charcot restraint orthotic walker (CROW)

The CROW is a bespoke, bivalved walker. They are extremely effective but expensive and time consuming to make. A CROW is used as an alternative to the total contact cast and, long term, for unstable ankles and feet that cannot be successfully accommodated in AFOs.

■ Knee scooter

This is a scooter with a shelf for the patient to kneel on so that the affected foot and ankle are entirely offloaded. They are used when total offloading is essential, as, for example, when interior fixation of a Charcot's osteoarthropathy has been performed and the patient cannot weightbear, or for patients who have indolent ulceration and really must not walk at all. It is important to ensure that the patient's eyesight is adequate to balance the scooter safely.

▨ Bed rest (heel protection is essential for high-risk patients on bed rest)

Occasionally, it is essential to keep the patient confined to bed with the feet elevated, as in cases of severe infection, following surgery, during the bony destructive phase of Charcot's osteoarthropathy when other methods are not suitable, or when other offloading methods have failed. However, it is difficult to find hospital beds unless the patient is acutely ill, and problems associated with bed rest include development of osteoporosis, thrombosis, depression, boredom, and bedsores.

OFFLOADING MANAGEMENT PROGRAMMES

▨ For patients at Stage 1 (low-risk foot)

The main aim is to maintain the feet in a healthy state and to prevent future foot problems by selecting the appropriate size and style of shoes and providing education programmes explaining how unsuitable foot wear damages the feet and leads to future problems. Almost all diabetic feet at Stage 1 (without deformity, oedema or callus) can be accommodated in high-street footwear.

▨ For patients at Stage 2 (high-risk foot)

Patients at this stage will have neuropathy and some will also have ischaemia, deformity, oedema, callus, Charcot feet and/or healed ulcers. The aim is to prevent ulceration while enabling the patient to lead as normal a life as possible (Fig. 4.8).

Footwear advice is needed by many patients: however, those without deformity, oedema, limited joint mobility or callus, and with no history of ulceration, can wear off-the-shelf shoes and do not need to be referred to the podiatrist or the orthotist.

Diabetic feet in the higher stages, including some at Stage 2, may be extremely complex biomechanically and subjected to high pressure and frictional and shearing forces, which will lead to callus, blistering, and ulceration if not relieved. Patients in Stage 2 can suffer from the following problems:

- neuropathy
- ischaemia
- previous history of ulcer
- fibrofatty padding depletion

- deformity
- oedema
- callus/corns.

They might need:

- orthotics
- ready-made, off-the-shelf stock shoes, trainer-style sports shoes or mountain boots
- extra-depth lace-ups
- modular shoes or footwear adaptations
- bespoke footwear (Fig. 4.9).

Fig. 4.8 (A) Thong sandals are widely worn in developing countries. This patient from Sri Lanka has developed interdigital ulceration to her first and second toes, where the thong has rubbed her foot. (B) This sandal was developed by the podiatry service in Singapore, to produce a safer alternative to thong sandals, for use in tropical climates. The velcro straps are adjustable, and the sole is thick enough to prevent puncture injuries from stepping on nails.

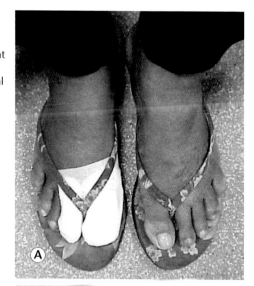

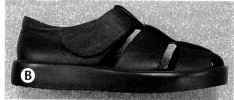

Fig. 4.9 These bespoke shoes are sufficiently long, broad and deep to accommodate deformity and contain a cradled insole. However, they are not fashionable and many patients refuse to wear them.

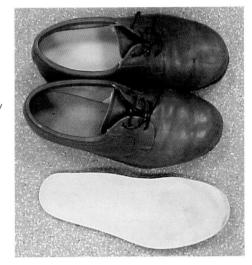

A few patients at Stage 2, with severe deformity, Charcot's osteoarthropathy, or a long history of relapse of ulceration, may need to wear CROWs or AFOs long term.

Many patients with long-term neuropathy have poor proprioception and some have postural hypotension. Many neuroischaemic patients are elderly and frail. Unsteady patients may benefit from a walking stick, crutch, Zimmer frame or wheelchair. Patients with neuroischaemic feet benefit from cushioned insoles and extra depth, wide fitting shoes.

The size and style of shoes needs careful selection. Very high-risk patients with previous ulceration or a history of relapse may need to agree to undertake limited walking, taking short steps in special footwear as described below, and should, wherever possible, avoid areas of employment that require long hours of walking, standing or driving, which are not suitable for diabetic foot patients. Activity monitoring may be useful in patients with recurrent foot problems. David Armstrong has described a device for this, but it is extremely expensive.

Other suitable interventions for the stage 2 foot, which can improve outcomes, include:

- felt padding
- special education on fitting shoes: shoes should not be sent out to the patient by post even after the second fitting. they should be issued face to face with the patient
- regular shoe checks (at every clinic visit)
- regular inspections and repairs of footwear, both inside and outside, are important to detect rough or deformed or stretched areas or penetrating objects or foreign bodies (as part of a trauma prevention programme) (Fig. 4.10)
- socks (incorporating silicone, or padded sports socks: there should be no prominent seams or tight elastic round ankle).

■ For patients at Stage 3 (ulcerated foot)

All patients with current ulceration need special offloading footwear, casts or other devices to reduce pressure as described above, including:

- crutches
- Zimmer frame or similar device (some are fitted with wheels, some with a shelf to support the knee)
- wheelchair with plank to elevate foot
- electric cart or buggy
- total contact cast
- windowed wound protection cast
- removable bivalved cast
- Scotchcast boot

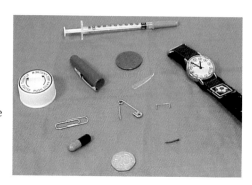

Fig. 4.10 All these objects were found in the shoes of neuropathic patients attending a diabetic foot clinic. Patients should always shake out their shoes before putting them on.

- Aircast products
- PRAFO
- AFO
- Patellar–tendon-bearing weight-relieving orthosis (PTB)
- CROW
- knee scooter
- bed rest (with heel protection).

Patients with ulcers should be strongly advised not to walk unless it is unavoidable and carefully educated to overcome the common perception that a wound that is not painful is not serious. For patients who insist that they must keep on the move, the most effective offloading techniques include:

- crutches
- Zimmer frame
- total contact cast
- Scotchcast boot
- CROW
- electric cart or buggy
- wheelchair.

To achieve optimal effective offloading, the podiatrist should make enquiries about the patient's lifestyle and activities to select the most suitable offloading device and also to see if it is feasible to reduce the amount of walking.

■ For patients at Stage 4 (infected foot)

Patients with current infection need complete offloading of the affected foot with:

- bedrest
- crutches
- wheel chair with plank to elevate foot.

Education is needed to explain that walking on an infected foot will cause great danger that the infection will spread and destroy the foot.

A Zimmer or crutches or wheelchair should be used if essential, but the foot should be kept off the ground. Once the infection has cleared the patient can enter the Stage 3 management programme described above.

■ For patients at Stage 5 (necrotic foot)
Wet necrosis
Patients with wet necrosis should initially be on bedrest and have intravenous antibiotics and surgery. Postsurgery, if still infected, they enter the Stage 4 offloading programme. When it is sure that infection is under control, they are managed as at Stage 3 until healing is achieved, and then at Stage 2 long term. Following a minor amputation, rehabilitation should be gradual because overloading the recovering foot may lead to development of an acute Charcot's osteoarthropathy.

Dry necrosis
Patients with dry necrosis awaiting autoamputation should be accommodated in a Scotchcast boot or Darco sandal and walk as little as possible. Wheelchairs should be used for essential movements.

FURTHER CONSIDERATIONS WHEN SELECTING OFFLOADING DEVICES
Podiatrists should be aware that the offloading advice that they give may conflict with the management of the patient's diabetes or other health conditions. For example, lack of exercise can make patients gain weight and render the diabetes harder to control. Physiotherapists are often concerned about muscle atrophy and joint contractures when elderly frail patients are not encouraged to walk.

■ Offloading for research studies
Pressure relief in research studies needs to be as uniform as possible, so that the true effect of the aspect of wound care being studied can be truly assessed.

■ Surgery
Although surgery can be helpful in some cases when excessive mechanical forces are due to structural abnormalities, rapid access to orthopaedic surgeons is a problem in many areas of the United Kingdom where there are not enough specialist foot and ankle surgeons. Increasingly, podiatric surgeons are filling the gap but many practitioners are reluctant to refer high-risk diabetic feet to

them. Furthermore, some of the feet that might in theory benefit from surgery are in practice extremely high risk by virtue of profound neuropathy, osteopenia, ischaemia, and reluctance of the patient to follow advice.

Surgery to improve offloading is usually only undertaken in Stage 1 feet or neuropathic feet. Before considering surgery for the neuroischaemic foot, it is necessary to correct ischaemia with angioplasty or bypass, and following vascular intervention only essential procedures should be undertaken because ischaemia can deteriorate again before healing has been achieved.

For the neuropathic foot, surgery can sometimes achieve very good results.

Case study

A 46-year-old female patient with type 1 diabetes of 23 years duration and intractable neuropathic ulceration underwent a modified Fowler's procedure with removal of the 2nd, 3rd, 4th and 5th metatarsal heads through dorsal incisions and remained ulcer free for 17 years.

Procedures include:

- Exostectomy: this is a very successful procedure for offloading plantar ulceration of a rocker-bottom Charcot foot, where any bony prominence underlying the ulcer is removed and shaved smooth.
- Severely deformed or unstable Charcot feet may be improved by surgery. These are major procedures and should not be performed during the acute phase of bony destruction, but delayed until the foot has settled down (see Chapter 7).
- Correction of hammer toe.
- Correction of mallet toe.
- Correction of claw toes.
- Excision of sesamoids.
- Excision of metatarsal heads.
- Osteotomy.
- Achilles tendon lengthening.

Problems associated with surgery to high-risk neuropathic feet to offload pressure include:

- increased rates of infection
- poor wound healing
- failed wound healing
- initiation of Charcot's osteoarthropathy.

Careful follow up is always needed.

FURTHER ASPECTS OF OFFLOADING TO BE CONSIDERED

Podiatrists should try to be imaginative about offloading. With modern technology there is no reason why patients should be confined to the house and unable to get outside. House adaptations, such as fitting stair lifts and ramps, will often be less expensive than moving house. The need for offloading should usually not prevent patients from working: firms over a certain size have quotas for disabled people. Nor are all forms of exercise absolutely vetoed: swimming is possible with cast protectors and upper limb exercising with weights, or other non-weight-bearing exercises. An exercise bicycle may be used if care is taken not to apply pressure to the ulcerated part of the foot.

It should not be forgotten that the effect of inactivity, leading to loss of fitness, may be a contributing factor to higher mortality rates in people with diabetic foot complications.

OFFLOADING BED-BOUND DIABETIC PATIENTS

Bed-bound patients, especially if they are frail and largely immobile, are at high risk of developing pressure ulcers. Special pressure-relieving mattresses and regular turning are helpful. Problems may be caused by:

- eating in bed and spilling crumbs; lying on crumbs can cause tissue breakdown
- lying on other foreign objects in the bed
- course-textured or wrinkled sheets
- sliding down the bed so that the feet are pressing against the foot-board of the bed.

Patients will need help moving up and down the bed because unassisted attempts can cause frictional injuries to the heels.

Antithrombotic tights can lead to nail problems unless the area covering the toes is folded back.

OFFLOADING THE PODIATRIST

It is not only the diabetic foot which needs to be offloaded; podiatrists are also vulnerable to overloading – of hands, wrists, arms, back, and neck. Overstrain injuries and repetitive stresses are common in the profession. It is important for podiatrists to be aware of the early signs of problems so that these can be treated or corrected. Some podiatrists regularly wear a splint or neck brace at work to prevent a problem from becoming intractable.

Good posture is important, as is having a good operator's chair, with wheels, which is set at a suitable height. Podiatrists should refuse to use poor quality, stiff instruments, or to treat more patients than is possible safely and healthily in a session. As a rule of thumb, a podiatrist should not agree to offer more than nine 'full treatments' of high-risk diabetic patients per session: for new patients, even more time per patient should be allocated.

The height and tilt of the patient's chair, and the position of the leg rests, should be adjusted frequently to ensure that, as different areas of the foot are worked on, the position is always optimal for the operator.

Podiatrists should obtain training in manual handling of patients and follow the rules and guidelines. In high-risk clinics, a hoist is a very useful piece of equipment.

Podiatrists who are injured at work should always fill in an accident form, try to learn from the experience, and seek help from the occupational health department if problems arise.

5 The infected foot

…Burns under feigned ashes,
And will at last break out into a flame:
As fester'd members rot, but by degree,
Till bones and flesh and sinews fall away.

William Shakespeare, Henry VI Part I. III. I. 189

Infection is the great destroyer of the diabetic foot. It is rarely the primary cause of ulceration but it is quick to take advantage of any breaches in the mantle of diabetic skin. Sometimes infection appears to have entered the foot through microscopic breaks, and it is hard to locate the primary portal of entry. Infection can invade the diabetic foot:

- Through intact but macerated callus or skin.
- Through broken skin.
- By secondarily infecting tinea pedis, blisters, or burns.
- Through tissues subjected to pressure from a thickened nail plate or callus.
- Injected deep into the foot by a puncture wound from, say, a tack or nail that penetrates the sole of the shoe before entering the foot.
- Very rarely, infection presents as a blood borne infection that has spread to a site far distant from a foot ulcer, or which has spread to the foot from a distant site.

INFECTION IS USUALLY A SECONDARY COMPLICATION OF FOOT ULCER

Infection of the diabetic foot presents most frequently as a complication of ulcers that were primarily caused by:

- neuropathy
- ischaemia
- trauma.

131

■ Effect of autonomic neuropathy on susceptibility to infection

The protective skin mantle may become more permeable as a result of autonomic neuropathy, with reduced sweating, subsequent drying of the skin, and resulting fissure formation, thus rendering the foot more susceptible to infection and providing portals of entry for invading microorganisms.

■ Effect of poor metabolic control on susceptibility to infection

Survival and multiplication of microorganisms is often easier in a sugar-rich diabetic environment. White cells might function less efficiently in hyperglycaemia.

■ Effect of sensory neuropathy on susceptibility to infection

Whatever the mode of entry, having invaded the diabetic foot with neuropathy, infection can spread with alarming rapidity. This is probably because pain is diminished or absent, so the patient often fails to seek treatment and continues to walk. With every step, infection is pumped through the foot.

People with protective pain sensation hobble and limp even when a foot injury is slight but profound neuropaths continue to walk and bear weight on an infected foot even when the foot is almost destroyed: there is little pain and little loss of function.

There may be further subtle effects of neuropathy on the inflammatory process and the body's ability to fight infection.

■ Effect of ischaemia on the foot's ability to fight infection

An effective inflammatory response is not possible in the absence of a good blood supply. Much of the inflammatory response to injury or infection depends on increased blood flow to the tissues and, in severe ischaemia, this is not possible. Ischaemia also makes it harder to diagnose infection, as there may be absence of warmth, swelling, and redness even if severe infection is present.

■ Effects of foot anatomy on infection

When infection occurs within a tightly bound foot compartment, swelling cannot be accommodated and leads to local ischaemia followed by necrosis.

THE NATURAL HISTORY OF DIABETIC FOOT INFECTION

The natural history of infection in the diabetic foot usually begins with a break in the skin, which may be followed by:

- healing failure
- local infection
- spreading infection
- severe life- and/or limb-threatening infection.

It is difficult to predict which wounds will heal quickly, with no trouble, and which wounds will fail to heal and ultimately develop infection. Few laboratories offer quantitative microbiology, but if this was available then increased numbers of organisms within a wound might be related to healing failure and potential to develop invasive infection. Within wounds, some microorganisms are embedded within a protective biofilm, removal of which (wound bed preparation) might kick-start healing; this might be one of the reasons why neuropathic ulcers respond well to vigorous debridement.

■ Healing failure

The wound does not appear to be overtly infected but fails to respond to good wound management and offloading. A swab or tissue sample should be sent for microscopy and culture, and the patient should be reviewed by a multidisciplinary team.

■ Local infection (some or all of the following are present)
(Fig. 5.1)

Fig. 5.1 Increased moisture and discharge are early warning signs of infection. A swab from this ulcer grew *Staphylococcus aureus* and beta haemolytic streptococcus.

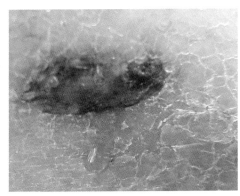

- Wound bed discoloration.
- Change in texture of wound bed surface.
- Increased moisture of wound bed.
- Increased discharge.
- Local cellulitis (around ulcer) ≤2 cm.
- Swelling.
- Warmth.

These patients need oral antibiotics and should be reviewed by a multidisciplinary team within 1 week.

■ **Spreading infection (some or all of the following are present)** (Fig. 5.2)

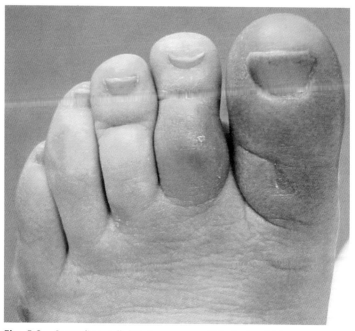

Fig. 5.2 Spreading cellulitis in a neuropathic foot, which was detected at a routine clinic appointment for nail cutting. The patient had no symptoms and was unaware that anything was wrong.

- Soft tissue infection with sloughy wound bed.
- Spreading cellulitis ≥2 cm.
- Purulent discharge.
- Lymphangitis.
- Lymphadenitis.
- Pain.

These patients need intramuscular or intravenous antibiotics and benefit from hospital admission. If admission is not possible, the patient should be seen daily by the community nurse or podiatrist.

■ Severe life- and/or limb-threatening infection (some or all of the following are present) (Fig. 5.3)

- Blue black discoloration.
- Breakdown and sloughy liquefaction of tissue.
- Tissue necrosis.
- Gas in the tissues.
- Fever, malaise, fatigue, rigors, and 'flu-like' symptoms.
- Septicaemia.

These patients need intravenous antibiotics and usually need surgical debridement. Hospital admission is essential and the foot should be inspected twice daily. If the infection is not controlled then the infection will end with major amputation or death.

DIFFICULTIES IN STAGING INFECTIONS

Staging infections is a useful, practical clinical tool only when each stage is a distinct clinical entity requiring a distinct management programme. However, in practice, staging diabetic foot infection has its limitations because, in the diabetic foot, it can often be very difficult to assess the boundaries of infection and determine which stage of infection is present. Furthermore, it seems that infection can deteriorate very rapidly and patients can move from one stage to another in a very short time.

When neuropathy and ischaemia are present, the symptoms and signs of infection are masked and what is apparently a mild infection can be very difficult to control. The boundaries between local, spreading, and severe infections might not be distinct and there may be areas of overlap. To overcome this difficulty, it is very important

Fig. 5.3 Severe infection in a neuroischaemic foot. (A) Note the bluish discoloration at the apex of the toe and the mucky, sloughy appearance of the small ulcer just proximal to the nail. The patient was admitted for intravenous antibiotics. (B) The dark area is a cavity filled with gas. Crepitus was evident when the foot was palpated.

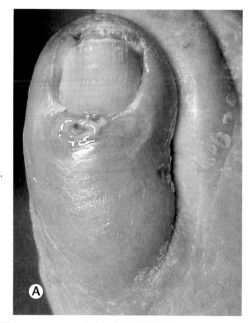

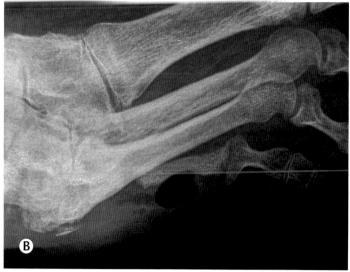

for podiatrists to be aware that if microbiological control is lost the foot can move from one stage of infection to another within a few hours. It is, therefore, essential to review infected feet regularly and frequently (preferably on a daily basis) and to adopt a 'worst-case scenario' in cases where the stage is unclear or the foot is not responding to treatment. 'When in doubt, assume the worst' is an important adage for diabetic foot infection management.

OTHER SYSTEMS FOR STAGING INFECTIONS, AND USING GUIDELINES

To describe foot infections in a useful way that can be used as a framework for care, other staging systems for infection in the diabetic foot have been developed by local, national, and international groups, including the American Diabetes Association and the International Consensus Group on the Diabetic Foot. Most groups have suggested that diagnosis of infection should depend on the presence of two or more of the usual signs and symptoms that accompany infection, namely:

- fever
- raised white blood cell count
- induration (hardening)
- oedema
- purulent discharge
- cellulitis extending more than 2 cm.

However, as already emphasized, some of these signs and symptoms of infection might be absent in the diabetic foot patient. Systemic signs, such as fever and raised white cell count, are absent in 50% of diabetic patients with severe infections. Purulent discharge is an unreliable sign if an ulcer is sealed off with callus, when purulent discharge will only be evident after debridement has enabled the infection to drain.

Despite these problems, there is clear opinion among existing consensus groups and infectious disease specialists that infection must always be diagnosed clinically and not microbiologically, and that antibiotics should very rarely be used in the absence of two or more of the above signs and symptoms.

Unfortunately, although these rigid criteria may be very effective in managing infections in other areas, they do not seem to work as well for diabetic foot patients as for non-diabetic patients. This might be because the signs and symptoms included do not take into account the unique combinations of peripheral neuropathy, peripheral vascular disease, and a compromised immune system in diabetic foot patients, which may render the usual signs and symptoms of infection unreliable.

It might also be the case that, when signs and symptoms of infection are present in a diabetic foot, they are markers or indicators of a degree of infection that is far more dangerous than an apparently similar degree of infection in a non-diabetic, sensate foot in a patient who has no peripheral vascular disease and is not immunosuppressed. It is essential that podiatrists and all healthcare professionals realize that diabetic foot infections are frequently much more severe than surface appearances suggest. This is sometimes called 'iceberg foot' because when an iceberg floats on the sea, around seven-tenths of its bulk are hidden from sight below the surface.

Guidelines and rules are useful only if they are:

- based on hard evidence, preferably from sufficiently large randomized clinical trials
- written by a group of experienced and open-minded clinicians with extensive clinical experience
- reliable.

Bad guidelines can be used to constrain clinicians and following them blindly can have a deleterious result. Guidelines are unlikely to improve outcomes for the diabetic foot unless those who draw them up accept that they are dealing with a unique entity by virtue of:

- microbiological flora
- immunological status
- the presence of neuropathy or neuroischaemia.

Current guidelines drawn up for the diagnosis and management of the diabetic foot do not differ greatly from guidelines for the management of infection in non-diabetic patients. Outcomes in diabetic patients treated according to existing guidelines are poor.

Modern medicine is obsessive about producing guidelines. Dr Rhys Williams, an epidemiologist, has described 'evidence-based paralysis', a situation when clinicians become afraid to base judgements on long clinical experience where evidence from randomized clinical trials is lacking.

THE CLINICIAN'S DILEMMA

There seems to be little doubt, anecdotally, that many infections in diabetic feet heal quickly, with or without treatment, and never lead to severe problems. However, there are no reliable statistics to reveal how often this occurs, nor is there any way for the clinician to tell at the start which patients will do well and which badly.

Any podiatrist who works in a diabetic foot clinic for high-risk patients, and offers an emergency service for diabetic foot patients in trouble, will see a great many diabetic feet with severe uncontrolled infections. Sometimes there is extensive tissue damage and feet take many months to heal. Sometimes a patient reaches the diabetic foot clinic too late and the only possible treatment is a major amputation. Often, patients report that the problem began with a 'little thing'; that they pulled off a piece of loose skin or applied a proprietary or folk remedy to a crack or blister or callus, or ignored a small problem because it did not hurt. Others have no idea how or why the problem arose.

Podiatrists working with diabetic foot patients need to take all foot injuries and all foot infections extremely seriously and should be guided in their work by the following alarming statistics:

- people with diabetes comprise at least 50% of all major amputations
- 85% of these amputations begin with a foot ulcer
- infection is nearly always involved in the final common pathway to amputation.

These statistics are ignored at the clinician's – and the patient's – peril. The author has spent most of her working life in a diabetic foot clinic working with a physician who also regarded infection as the great destroyer of the diabetic foot and was always concerned to detect infection early and treat it aggressively. She has talked to many podiatric colleagues who came to work at King's on a training rotation but also worked for part of the week in other situations where they found it difficult to obtain antibiotics for diabetic patients with foot infections. These visiting podiatrists welcomed having rapid access to antibiotics for patients with infections at the hospital clinic, and said that ulcers healed more quickly when antibiotics were available. This is consistent with the author's own experience.

THE USEFULNESS OF MICROBIOLOGY

It is commonly stated that microbiology should not be used to diagnose infection, that swabs should not be sent to the laboratory unless infection is suspected and that the purpose of microbiology is to guide choice of antibiotic therapy. However, a positive wound swab may be a useful warning of impending infection. A small study at King's, which followed 64 diabetic foot patients with apparently clean ulcers and no signs or symptoms of infection, found that the majority of patients who subsequently developed foot infections had a positive wound swab at entry to the study.

However, it is important for podiatrists to be open-minded and look to the published evidence and existing guidelines, as well as at first-hand experiences of coping with diabetic foot infections. As is the case with many aspects of the role of the podiatrist, there is a disconcerting dearth of evidence on which to ground firm assertions relating to management of infection.

Experienced podiatrists are aware of how rapidly things can go wrong with a diabetic foot, and how an apparently clean, granulating wound, can develop devastating infection almost overnight. Seeing patients week by week and year by year, we also observe that a severe bout of infection can retard wound healing for many weeks, and that patients who are healing well on antibiotics will often quickly relapse and develop fresh infection within a few days of stopping antibiotics.

When podiatrists are working in inner city areas of great social deprivation, where poverty and ignorance are great barriers to care, it can be extremely difficult to persuade patients who lack protective pain sensation to take infection seriously, inspect their feet regularly, and act quickly on the early signs that infection is developing. It is for this reason, that many healthcare practitioners in the field of diabetic foot care believe that diabetic foot patients need protection with prophylactic antibiotics.

WHEN MIGHT PROPHYLACTIC ANTIBIOTICS BE CONSIDERED?

The approach that uses prophylactic antibiotics might be applied to:

- Elderly patients who live in conditions of poverty and social deprivation and may have problems accessing care.

- Ischaemic patients.
- Patients in end-stage renal failure.
- Immunosuppressed patients (e.g. those on steroids).
- Patients with previous history of frequent severe foot problems and/or foot infections.
- Major amputees whose remaining foot is very precious.
- Patients who are unable or unwilling (often through no fault of their own) to look after themselves and take full responsibility for their health.

The last set of patients should not be judged too harshly: they may have poor vision, lack of protective pain sensation, and low expectations.

GANGRENE IS A DISEASE OF THE POOR

Affluent and well-educated patients who understand the importance of taking an interest in their own health and playing an active part in management decisions are far less vulnerable to overwhelming infection. 'Gangrene', said the great American diabetologist, Eliott Joslin, 'is a disease of the poor'. Even for affluent patients, neuropathy is an all-pervading danger: it makes the world a hostile place, but patients who tend to be more demanding and to seek help earlier seem to have better outcomes.

'NEUROPATHY OF THE BRAIN'

Neuropathy sometimes seems to affect the patient's grey matter as well as the feet; some diabetic patients develop devastating infections time after time, yet seem to be incapable of:

- understanding that they are in danger
- learning what they need to do to keep themselves safe
- following the simplest instructions.

Following a sharp experience, say, loss of a toe due to infection, these patients seem to accept that they will need to take special care of their feet in future. But after a short time they return to their old ways and it is as if the previous episode had never occurred. And the next time they develop a foot problem and an infection they again fail to seek help 'because it didn't hurt'.

Decisions about whether to ask for antibiotics for a particular patient will, therefore, often depend on the previous history of the patient. Some individuals seem to have a particular susceptibility to infections, and others seem to be incapable of taking care of their ulcerated feet and detecting infection early

DIAGNOSIS OF INFECTION

■ Diagnosing infection early
The podiatrist should examine the foot carefully, searching for:

- swelling
- warmth
- pain or throbbing
- open lesions
- discharge
- colour change of skin or wound bed.

Other signs of infection include:

- a pouting wound, surrounded by tightly bound-down callus with a slit-like sinus aperture that probes deeply
- a 'soupy' look
- increased wetness of the wound
- slimy quality of associated slough and soft tissues
- blue or purple discolouration
- blebs or blistering near the ulcer
- tracking of fluid under callus (Fig. 5.4)
- tracking of the ulcer beneath surrounding skin
- crepitus in the tissues.

The help of other members of the diabetic foot team should be sought earlier rather than later if the podiatrist detects the above signs and symptoms.

■ Diagnosing osteomyelitis
When diagnosing osteomyelitis the following are useful:

- X-ray (Fig. 5.5)
- probing to bone
- detection of 'sausage toe' (Fig. 5.6).

Fig. 5.4 Beneath the plaque of callus is an infected neuropathic ulcer. Pus from the ulcer is tracking beneath the skin.

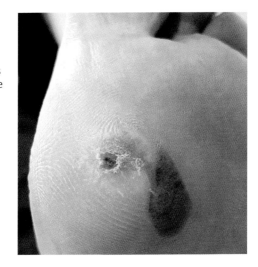

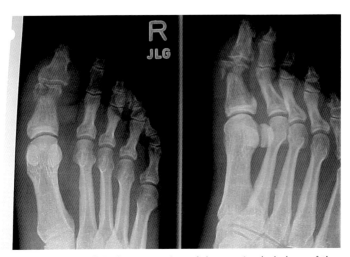

Fig. 5.5 Osteomyelitis: fragmentation of the proximal phalanx of the great hallux.

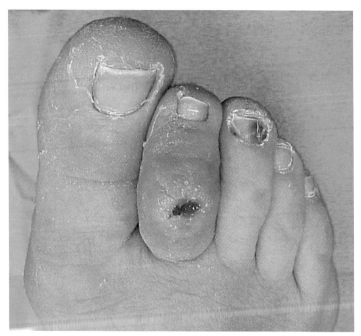

Fig. 5.6 Osteomyelitis: 'sausage toe', with red, fusiform swelling. The small ulcer on the dorsum of the toe probed to bone.

TREATING INFECTION IN THE DIABETIC FOOT

The aim is to:

- control the infection
- prevent deterioration
- heal the foot as soon as possible.

■ Debriding the infected foot

Infected diabetic feet need debridement. The aim is to:

- remove all overlying and surrounding callus and non-viable tissue so that the true dimensions of the problem can be clearly seen
- drain pus.

Diabetic feet do not tolerate the presence of necrotic tissue and pus under pressure and deteriorate very rapidly in these circumstances.

Even if the patient is about to be admitted to hospital, it is useful for samples to be taken in the diabetic foot clinic by the podiatrist and sent immediately to the laboratory so as to avoid delay in identifying the microorganisms involved. Samples of pus or deep tissue (discard surface tissue) may be sent to the microbiologists for microscopy and culture. Table 5.1 may assist practitioners in deciding the extent of debridement needed.

If the foot is neuropathic then any discoloured areas of the wound bed should be debrided; sinuses should be probed, and laid open where possible; and surrounding undermined skin should be removed.

Table 5.1 *Different appearances of normal and infected dead tissues*

	Normal	*Infected or dead*
Bone		
Colour	Ivory	Yellow, brown black
Consistency	Hard and firm	Crumbly, soft, with loose bits attached
Texture	Smooth	Rough
Bleeds	Yes	No
Skin and soft tissue		
Colour	Pink*	Red, purple, blue, brown, black, pale
Consistency	Firm, resilient	Flaccid, slack, blistered
Texture	Smooth	Slimy
Bleeds	Yes	No
Tendon		
Colour	Yellow/cream	White, black
Bleeds	No	No
Slough		
Consistency	Firm	Very loose and slippery
Smell	No	Yes

*Allowances should of course be made for colour differences in the skin of people of different races.

If the foot is ischaemic and infection is suspected, then advice should be sought from the vascular surgeons regarding the extent of debridement. (In both cases, if the patient subsequently goes for surgical debridement it should be mandatory for surgical debridings to be sent from the operating theatre to the laboratory.)

■ Dressing the infected diabetic foot

After debridement the wound should be cleaned with normal saline and dressed with a sterile non-adherent dressing, which can be easily lifted for wound inspection. Ideally, the dressing should be held in place with a tubular bandage, which can accommodate swelling, and the foot should be inspected regularly to ensure that the bandage is not too tight. If exudate strikes through dressing and bandage then these need to be replaced.

■ Marking extent of cellulitis

It is helpful to assess whether cellulitis is spreading by tracing the area of cellulitis with a spirit-based pen. The foot should then be examined regularly to see whether cellulitis has spread beyond the marked area.

■ Seeking to improve the blood supply

If the pedal pulses cannot be palpated, and further studies indicate that the foot is ischaemic, then the advice of the vascular team should be sought urgently. Ischaemic feet cannot mount a good inflammatory response to fight infection and delay in treatment of ischaemia may result in loss of a limb that was potentially salvageable.

■ Offloading the infected foot

Patients with foot infections should be strongly advised not to walk and to keep the foot elevated.

MICROORGANISMS AND THE DIABETIC FOOT

Microorganisms associated with diabetic foot infections include:

- Gram-positives: including *Staphylococcus aureus*, *Streptococcus* and *Enterococcus* species
- Anaerobes: including *Bacteroides*, *Clostridium*, *Peptostreptococcus* and *Peptococcus* species

- Gram-negatives: including *Klebsiella*, *Escherichia coli*, *Enterobacter*, *Pseudomonas*, *Citrobacter*, *Morganella morganii*, *Serratia*, *Acinetobacter*, and *Proteus* species.

Many microorganisms, such as *Streptococcus milleri*, can cause tissue necrosis in the diabetic foot but rarely cause problems in patients who are not diabetic and not immunocompromised. However, it may be possible to predict the likely infecting organisms from a variety of clues, including the:

- nature of the patient
- nature of the wound (neuropathic or ischaemic)
- past history of the patient
- local environment
- duration of the wound (acute or chronic)
- previous antibiotics used to treat the patient
- patient's history of recent hospital admissions.

All of the above may render the presence of certain organisms more likely. The practitioner can generalize that in an acute wound in a neuropath with no previous history of foot problems, *Staphylococcus aureus* and group B streptococci are the more likely organisms. Anaerobes thrive in ischaemic tissue. Patients with previous history of antibiotic treatment may be more prone to have polymicrobial infections. Recent hospital admissions make infection with methicillin-resistant *Staphylococcus aureus* (MRSA) more likely. However, it is dangerous to rely too much on speculation, guesswork, or over-generalisation when the patient is at high risk and the consequences of making a wrong decision are dire. In these circumstances it may be wise initially to cover a wide spectrum of organisms and to narrow down the antibiotics given after results from microscopy and culture have been obtained.

■ Making decisions

The situations that affect decision making are discussed in further detail below. The podiatrist should consider the following aspects.

The nature of the patient

- Elderly or frail or immunocompromised?
- Can the patient be relied on to detect problems early and return to clinic promptly if deterioration occurs?

- Will the patient follow advice?
- Can the patient perform self-care? If not, a nurse should be asked to visit.

The nature of the wound

- Is the ulcer neuropathic or neuroischaemic?
- Is the ulcer superficial or deep?
- Was the problem associated with a puncture wound?

The past history of the patient

- Has the patient a previous history of severe foot infections?
- Is the patient at particularly high risk by virtue of renal disease or immunosuppression?
- Have problems arisen in the past because of non-compliance?

The local environment

- Does the patient live at home?
- Is the patient socially isolated?
- Does the patient have adequate support?
- Is the patient cared for by others?

The duration of the wound

Is the wound acute or chronic? Acute wounds are more likely to contain *Staphylococcus aureus* or group B streptococci. Chronic wounds are more likely to have polymicrobial infections with anaerobes and Gram-negatives.

Previous antibiotics used to treat the patient

Previous infection treatments may mean that useful results may be available.

- What were the previous microorganisms detected and antibiotics given and how did the patient respond?
- Is there a previous history of MRSA infection?

Whether there have been recent hospital admissions

Patients who have been in hospital may be more likely to suffer infections with MRSA or other resistant organisms.

■ Treating infections with antibiotics

Antibiotics may be delivered by the following routes:

● topical (not usually recommended for diabetic foot patients)
● oral
● intramuscular
● intravenous.

■ Organisms commonly found in diabetic foot infections

Organisms commonly found in diabetic foot infections are given below:

Staphylococcus aureus
Worldwide, this is the most common diabetic foot pathogen.

MRSA
This is now a common organism in many countries, and is resistant to flucloxacillin. Extended sensitivities should be asked for. MRSA can be treated with other oral agents (which should be given in combination as use of a single agent will rapidly develop resistance), with intramuscular teicoplanin, or with intravenous vancomycin.

Streptococcus groups A, B, C, E, F and G
There are several different groups of streptococcus, each of which is associated with different types of infection; group B is the most common. Group A streptococcus causes erysipelas. An infection with a streptococcus in combination with a staphylococcus can lead to a very serious, rapidly spreading infection because they are synergistic: the streptococcus produces hyaluronidase, which breaks down the tissues and assists in the spread of necrotising toxins produced by the staphylococcus.

Enterococcus
Enterococcus faecalis is rarely pathogenic. Vancomycin-resistant enterococcus (VSE) may cause problems in hospital patients.

Anaerobes
These are usually found in deep infections or chronic wounds. Clostridium perfringens causes gas gangrene.

Gram-negatives

Gram-negative bacteria can definitely be pathogenic and are often found in deep infections. *Pseudomonas aeruginosa* can betray its presence by a distinctive odour (fusty and mousy) and turquoise colour, which stains dressings (Fig. 5.7).

■ Use of antibiotics for the diabetic foot

Antibiotics for the diabetic foot may need to be started earlier, and continued for longer, than in corresponding conditions in non-diabetic feet, but there is no definite evidence as to optimal times to start and to stop antibiotics.

It is essential for the practitioner to try to weigh potential advantages against potential disadvantages to the individual patient and the general population. In practice, this can be very difficult to do, as podiatrists may feel that their duty is to their specific patient and not to a vague concept of future generations benefiting at the expense of current patients. Current guidelines on antibiotic use are of limited use for the practical management of high-risk diabetic foot patients.

When working with the high-risk diabetic foot, any microorganism can be a pathogen. Wherever antibiotics are used there is a potential for resistance in microorganisms to develop and spread. However, this is more likely if:

● inadequate doses are given
● patients do not finish the course

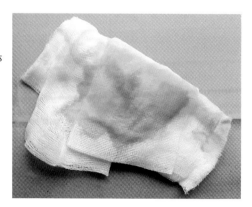

Fig. 5.7 The blue–green discoloration on this dressing was caused by *Pseudomonas aeruginosa*. The foot smelled musty, like mouse urine. The presence of pseudomonas was confirmed by microbiology.

- antibiotics are started and stopped very frequently
- animals are given prophylactic antibiotics
- aseptic and sterile procedures are inadequate
- infection control policies are inadequate or improperly policed.

◼ Infection control

It is important for podiatrists to be aware of the risks and to take special precautions to control the spread of infection from patient to podiatrist, from podiatrist to patient, and from patient to patient. Microorganisms are spread by:

- direct contact
- indirect contact: the hands of the podiatrist, patient contact surfaces, equipment, water
- airborne contact: dust, skin cells, skin squames, or bacterial spores.

Advanced age, diabetes, and vascular disease increase likelihood of infection. Care plans are essential for diabetic foot clinics to:

- identify infection hazards
- identify transmission risks
- reduce risk of transmission by taking standard precautions.

Standard precautions include:

- hand washing and hand rubbing with antiseptic gel
- use of protective clothing: aprons, gloves, masks, as appropriate
- preventing and managing sharps injuries
- safe disposal of clinical waste (which is contaminated with bodily fluids or human tissue)
- linen handling and processing
- instrument handling, decontamination and processing
- environmental cleaning
- clearing up of body fluid spillages
- aseptic techniques
- ensuring that material in direct contact with wound is sterile
- covering lesions on staff
- reporting accidents and taking steps to avoid recurrence
- managing eczema, dermatitis, etc. in staff and patients
- surveillance of cases of infection arising in patients of the diabetic foot clinic looking for patterns of infection and trends which might indicate problems with infection control.

Podiatrists performing sharp debridement of ulcers may be at risk from blood-borne viruses and should be immunized against the hepatitis B virus.

Individual care plans are needed and some patients may need to be treated with special precautions such as isolation.

Sometimes resistance to antibiotics can be passed from one organism to another.

▓ Antibiotic prescribing

A few podiatrists in the United Kingdom are now able to prescribe antibiotics for diabetic foot patients using patient group directives. However, most podiatrists do not prescribe and will need to request prescriptions from a physician. Nevertheless, it is important for podiatrists to be knowledgeable about antibiotics and their use. In particular, it is not fair for podiatrists to ask inexperienced doctors to prescribe specific drugs for a patient unless the podiatrist has carefully considered, in each individual case:

- what drug is most suitable
- what the potential problems might be
- whether the patient can tolerate it.

Although it is the doctor who is ultimately responsible for what he prescribes, the podiatrist also has a professional and moral obligation to weigh and consider the situation before making a request for specific antibiotics for a patient.

Oral antibiotics

Contraindications to specific antibiotics include:

- allergy
- possibility of drug interactions
- previous or current history of severe health problems associated with antibiotic use.

Common side effects include:

- rashes
- skin irritation
- pruritus
- loss of appetite
- nausea

- diarrhoea
- thrush.

Serious side effects of antibiotic use include:

- anaphylaxis
- Stevens–Johnson syndrome
- aplastic anaemia
- renal failure
- liver failure
- permanent deafness.

Patients should be warned to report any problems associated with antibiotic use immediately. Patients with moderate to severe nephropathy, end-stage renal failure, or impaired liver function, will need a reduced dose of many antibiotics, and some antibiotics that are known to be associated with kidney problems should never be used in renal patients. Liver function should be checked. Interactions between antibiotics and other drugs are common.

■ Antibiotic-related gastrointestinal problems

Many of the gastrointestinal (GI) problems associated with antibiotic use result from killing of the normal bowel flora. Patients on oral antibiotics should be advised to wash the tablets down with plenty of water, and to take products such as live yoghurt to recolonize the bowel and prevent stomach upsets. Nausea can be treated with drugs such as Maxolon®. A potentially life-threatening complication of antibiotic therapy is pseudomembranous colitis following overgrowth of the bowel with *Clostridium difficile*. This problem presents with pain and diarrhoea. Podiatrists should advise diabetic foot patients with antibiotic-associated diarrhoea to stop taking them and seek urgent review by an experienced physician.

■ Antibiotics delivered by intramuscular injection
Advantages

- Achieve higher levels of antibiotic than oral delivery.
- Less GI irritation.
- Avoid necessity of hospital admission for administration of intravenous antibiotics.

Associated problems

- Bruising and soreness at injection sites.
- Pain.
- Local fibrosis/sepsis.

A common contraindication to the use of intramuscular injections is concurrent treatment with warfarin.

In the United Kingdom, intramuscular drugs can be administered only by a trained healthcare professional. Patients report that it is very inconvenient if they have to wait at home for the nurse to call. However, patients with foot infections severe enough to warrant intramuscular antibiotics should be resting at home anyway.

■ Antibiotics delivered by intravenous route

These are usually given to hospital inpatients, via the arm veins, through a small venflon device. Associated problems include:

- phlebitis
- local pain and soreness.

Some centres are now delivering intravenous antibiotics to diabetic patients at home, often through a Hickman line, Pic line or central line.

■ Commonly used antibiotics

Details of some of the antibiotics commonly used to prevent or manage infections of the diabetic foot are listed below.

Amoxicillin

This can be delivered orally or intravenously and is effective against streptococci, including *Streptococcus faecalis*. However, it is unsuitable for patients with penicillin allergy.

Flucloxacillin

Delivered orally or intravenously. This is the ideal treatment for *Staphylococcus aureus* infection but cannot be used for patients with penicillin allergy.

Metronidazole

Delivered orally, intravenously, or per rectum. This is effective against anaerobes. When given orally it makes some patients feel very unwell.

Patients must be warned not to take alcohol when they are on metronidazole.

Ciprofloxacin

Oral or intravenous agent against Gram-negative organisms. Some patients complain of a metallic taste in the mouth. On rare occasions it makes patients hypoglycaemic (Ciproxin® was first investigated for its properties as a potential oral hypoglycaemic agent). Hallucinations were a problem with one patient, an elderly lady, who reported the presence of strange people dancing in her back garden every night. A problem was that she lived in an area of London where such capers were quite likely and it was several days before her daughter realized that the invaders were not real!

Erythromycin

An oral agent, useful against *Staphylococcus aureus* and streptococci for patients with penicillin allergy, but can cause severe gastrointestinal irritation. Patients on statins should temporarily stop them as erythromycin may increase the risk of myositis from statin therapy.

Clarithromycin

A very useful formulation of erythromycin, with far less gastrointestinal irritation. It needs to be taken only twice a day.

Fucidin® (fusidic acid)

Good bony penetration when given orally: effective against *Staphylococcus aureus* but should not be given alone as resistance will develop quickly. It should be accompanied by a further anti-staphylococcal agent.

Clindamycin

A useful oral antibiotic, active against staphylococci and streptococci, and also has anti-anaerobic activity. However, it has been associated with pseudomembranous colitis, which can be fatal. Patients on clindamycin who develop diarrhoea should stop taking the drug immediately and contact the person who prescribed it.

Rifampicin

Good oral anti-staphylococcal agent, with good bony penetration in cases of osteomyelitis, and is also active against streptococci.

Patients should be warned that it may colour urine red. Should not be given alone because resistance will develop rapidly. Should be used with a further anti-staphylococcal agent.

Trimethoprim

An oral agent that can be effective against moderate infections with MRSA when used in combination with one of the following: Fucidin®, rifampicin or doxycycline. Active against Gram-negative organisms.

Doxycycline

An oral agent that is tolerated well by renal patients.

Ceftriaxone

Given by intramuscular injection. Good against staphylococcus and streptococcus and Gram-negatives.

Teicoplanin

Given intramuscularly or intravenously. Active against Gram-positives, including MRSA. Extremely expensive and many GPs are reluctant to prescribe it.

Gentamicin

Given intravenously. Active against *Staphylococcus aureus*, coliforms and pseudomonas. Nephrotoxic – blood levels need to be checked regularly; ototoxic – one of the author's renal transplant patients, already blind from diabetic retinopathy, was rendered almost deaf as a result of treatment with gentamicin and Paul Brand described a similar case in a leprosy patient at Carville.

Vancomycin

Occasionally given orally to eliminate *Clostridium difficile* (see above), but usually given intravenously for severe infections. Effective against MRSA and enterococcus. Blood levels of vancomycin need to be checked regularly.

Piperacillin

Effective intravenous agent against coliforms and pseudomonas.

Linezolid
A new, and expensive antibiotic: effective against MRSA, but not yet licensed for the diabetic foot.

C reactive protein
When assessing a patient's response to treatment of severe infection, it is useful to look at serial measurement of C-reactive protein (CRP) as a measure of progress. Initially high levels of CRP that fall with treatment indicate that the treatment is working.

■ Unusual infections
Because diabetic patients are very prone to infection, they will sometimes present with unusual infections.

Case study

A 62-year-old man with type 2 diabetes and cirrhosis of the liver went to Florida on holiday and ate several raw oysters and clams in an oyster bar. He was not aware that within the Gulf of Florida an organism called *Vibrio vulnificus* infects oysters, which are harvested and then transported in unrefrigerated vans to oyster bars where they are served raw. The patient developed nausea, vomiting and diarrhoea, and a high fever. He was taken to the local emergency room, where he was found to be hypotensive and toxic. Fortunately his wife was able to give a history of imbibing raw oysters and the doctors in the emergency room were familiar with the signs and symptoms of *Vibrio vulnificus* and treated him immediately with an appropriate antibiotic. He was doubly susceptible, being immunocompromised by virtue of being diabetic and also having impaired liver function. He developed severe vasculitic lesions of the right hand and arm and both legs below the knee, resulting in destruction of epidermis.

He was flown back to the United Kingdom and his treatment consisted of intravenous antibiotics and flamazine dressings followed by split skin grafting.

Infections of the diabetic foot can spread with alarming rapidity.

Case study

A 42-year-old woman with type 2 diabetes of 3 years duration had a chronic onychocryptosis of the right hallux for 3 months which had not responded to conservative care. She underwent a partial right 1st nail avulsion with phenolization of the nail matrix late in the afternoon. The next morning when she woke she had slight pain and aching in the right thigh ('almost as if I had been kicked') and telephoned the foot clinic at 9.00 for advice.
She denied redness, swelling, pain or discharge in the right toe. She was asked to come to the clinic if the pain did not settle.
At 11.00 she felt weak, dizzy, and hot and her husband brought her to the diabetic foot clinic. She arrived at noon, carried in by her husband. The right foot and leg were grossly oedematous and red. She had a fever of 39°C and was hypotensive.
Our consultant, who carried a bleep, came to the foot clinic immediately, diagnosed septic shock, and admitted her for resuscitation and quadruple intravenous antibiotics. Blood cultures grew streptococcus but no growth was obtained from the toe. She eventually made a good recovery but needed to remain in hospital for 3 weeks.

Case study

In the early 1980s the author was asked to come up to the diabetic ward at King's to see a 60-year-old male carpenter with type 2 diabetes of 20 years duration. The patient was born in Jamaica and had not returned to his homeland for over 17 years. He had developed leg ulcers, which were treated by district nurses with dry dressings and bandaging for 9 months. He was admitted to hospital after developing rapid extension of ulceration, pain, and fever and it was noted that on both his lower legs, right knee and right forearm there were dark papules with central sinuses oozing dark oily fluid. He said that his leg ulcers had begun as similar papules.

Fluid was gently expressed from a papule and sent for microscopy and culture; fungal hyphae were reported but the species could not be determined. Samples of the organism were sent to mycological centres in the United Kingdom and abroad and an identification was finally made at Kew Gardens. The organism was *Plectophomella*, a fungus that usually infects elm trees. Only one other case of human infection with this particular fungus had ever been recorded.

In addition to this man's diabetes, he had a pre-leukaemic condition that might have rendered him more susceptible to infection.

Because the leg ulcers were so extensive and this case occurred in the 1980s, treatment options were limited and included the possibility of bilateral major amputation. He asked to go home for the weekend to consider his options, and committed suicide.

Case study

A 46-year-old woman with type 1 diabetes of 21 years duration bought a salicylic-acid-based callus remover and applied it to a callus on her left foot. Four days later she presented at the diabetic foot clinic as an emergency case with a painful foot. There was a macerated callus over her left 5th metatarsal head where the callus remover had been applied. The area was painful on direct pressure with surrounding cellulitis. Debridement revealed an abscess containing 4 mL of pus, which was drained, to expose an abscess cavity. Intramuscular antibiotics were prescribed and she returned in 3 days, spending the intervening period in bed at home with regular visits from the district nurse to administer the antibiotics and inspect the foot. The ulcer took 7 weeks to heal.

HOW TO TAKE SPECIMENS FROM AN ULCER

- The ulcer should first be sharp debrided.
- Clean the wound bed thoroughly by scrubbing it with sterile gauze moistened with saline.

- The wound bed is then gently but firmly scraped with a scalpel blade.
- The scrapings are sent for microscopy and culture in a sterile pot. The blade may be sent in the pot if prior agreement has been obtained from the laboratory.

Podiatrists who are worried about taking curettings in this way can rub the cleaned wound bed with a swab instead. The swab is then inserted into a tube of transport medium and sent to the laboratory.

Samples of tissue can also be taken from necrotic areas. The dry, surface tissue is first debrided away exposing the moist deeper tissues from which specimens are cut away.

Pus can be collected in a small sterile pot and sent to the laboratory.

OSTEOMYELITIS

The natural history of osteomyelitis is as follows. A break in the skin leads to:

- healing failure
- deepening of wound
- sloughy wound bed
- sinus formation
- sinus reaches bone or joint
- surface of bone becomes eroded
- infected bone dies and fragments.

If the affected area of bone involves a toe, then the toe takes on a red, sausage-like appearance with fusiform swelling.

Osteomyelitis is managed either by appropriate oral antibiotics, given for up to 3 months, or by surgery. Which option to choose may be a difficult decision, and will depend on the clinical appearance and the extent of bony changes on X-ray.

After bone has become infected it may take several weeks for this to show up on the X-ray.

INFECTION FOLLOWING PUNCTURE WOUNDS

Puncture wounds to the diabetic foot can lead to very severe infections and should always be taken seriously. American podiatrists Larry

Harkless, David Armstrong and colleagues working in the podiatry service at San Antonio, Texas, have described severe infections following puncture wounds:

- the punctures were initially regarded as trivial wounds
- *Pseudomonas aeruginosa* was the most commonly found organism
- the patients had been wearing training shoes.

In many puncture wounds the penetrating object has passed through the sole of the shoe and then injects microorganisms and foreign material deep into the foot. Often, the initial injury heals and seals in the infecting material. Discharge of pus is not possible and the foot suddenly develops catastrophic infection. Feet with puncture wounds should be X-rayed, treated with systemic antibiotics and observed very closely (Fig. 5.8).

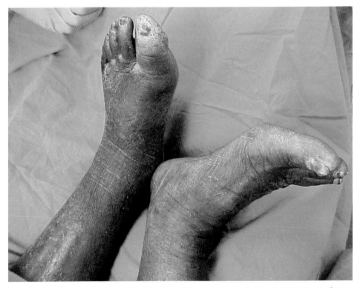

Fig. 5.8 A puncture wound has led to severe infection. Because the patient is Afro-Caribbean, with a pigmented skin, the cellulitis is not very easy to see unless the two feet are compared.

SYSTEMIC EFFECTS OF DIABETIC FOOT INFECTIONS

There is a suspicion that diabetic foot infection may destroy more than the foot. A recent study has indicated that patients with a history of foot infection with MRSA might be more likely to develop myocardial infarction, and that patients with foot infections that are apparently successfully treated may retain high levels of inflammation for several months after apparent clinical resolution of infection.

In summary, existing guidelines for the management of infection are more relevant to the management of the neuropathic foot than to the neuroischaemic foot, where following them can quickly result in catastrophe (Figs 5.9, 5.10).

However, it would be simplistic to say that the solution to the problem of the diabetic foot patient is always to provide antibiotics more frequently and for longer periods. Blanket prescriptions of antibiotics for all diabetic foot ulcers and injuries cannot be the solution to the problem of infection in the diabetic foot. The problems associated with too ready a use of antibiotics are that antibiotics are expensive and that side effects are common and may be severe.

There are also dangers of grooming microbial resistance. (The diabetic foot was recently described by an eminent North American

Case study

A 36-year-old man with type 2 diabetes mellitus and full-thickness wet necrosis extending from the tips of his toes to the bases of his metatarsal heads, only presented at the accident and emergency department after his girl friend told him his foot had 'turned green'. There was a heavy growth of pseudomonas with heavy exudates, which had stained callus green. He was Afro-Caribbean, with heavily pigmented skin, and his foot problem began when he trod on a nail at work. This punctured the sole of his shoe and entered his foot. He visited the GP who gave him a 5-day course of amoxicillin and did not offer a follow-up appointment. The foot appeared to heal fully, but 2 weeks later it had developed extensive wet necrosis. He had been told 2 years previously, in a hospital casualty department, that he had diabetes but had failed to keep a follow-up appointment or to seek care.

Fig. 5.9   A small ulcer on the 5th toe of this neuroischaemic foot had been caused by bathroom surgery. It was dressed every week by a community nurse but only referred on when the toe became gangrenous.

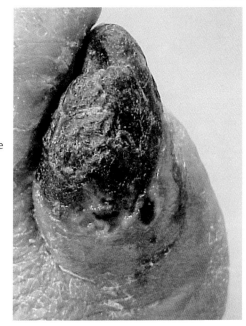

Fig. 5.10   This patient with neuropathy saw a community podiatrist regularly for debridement and dressings after developing a footwear-related blister. The ulcer did not heal, and was treated in the community for several months. The patient was only referred to the hospital diabetic foot clinic after infection developed, by which time the 'window of opportunity' to achieve rapid healing had closed. The toe was amputated.

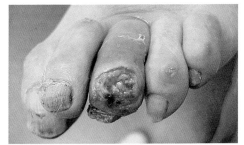

Case study

A 34-year-old man with type 2 diabetes of unknown duration developed paraesthesiae and found the tingling very annoying. He self-treated his problem by filling a bucket with boiling water from a kettle. He tested the water with his profoundly neuropathic big toe, decided that the temperature was acceptable, and soaked his feet in the bucket for several minutes, thus adding the problem of infected third-degree burns to his initial problem of a tingling, painful foot. He did not come to the hospital until the infection spread beyond the distribution of the neuropathy and his knees became painful. Five toes were amputated on each foot.

Case study

A 24-year-old man with type 1 diabetes of 9 years' duration went swimming in a local pool, hid his watch in his shoe, forgot that he had done so, and walked to the police station to report the theft of his watch. Three days later he discovered the watch in his shoe. He also found a large cavity in the plantar surface of his infected foot. When he presented at the diabetic foot clinic he had a severe infection with cellulitis extending to the knee, lymphangitis, and lymphadenitis. He was systemically unwell, with pyrexia of 38°C and rigors; he was not ketotic. We wished to admit him to hospital but he insisted on first telephoning his grandmother in Africa for advice. She said that he should on no account agree to enter hospital as 'people go to hospital to die'. However, he accepted intramuscular antibiotics, the foot was drained and debrided in the outpatient diabetic foot clinic, he attended daily for wound care, and the infection settled down. He returned to Africa before his foot was fully healed and was lost to follow up.

infectious disease specialist as 'a crucible for creating antibiotic resistance'.) The more antibiotics that are used, the greater the likelihood is that antibiotic resistance will develop, and antibiotic resistance is likely to become an enormous trouble, both for diabetic foot patients and for the population at large.

6 Management of vascular patients

We are all diseased,
And with our surfeiting and wanton hours,
Have brought ourselves into a burning fever,
And we must bleed for it …
… And purge the obstructions that begin to stop
Our very veins of life.

William Shakespeare, Henry IV Part II. IV. I. 65

The diabetic neuroischaemic foot is an unforgiving foot and, without expert, well-organized care, the outlook for patients is bleak. Most of the diabetic patients in the United Kingdom who undergo a major amputation are neuroischaemic. This is a specialist area of foot care and podiatrists should not work with these patients in isolation: they are sure to need help from other members of the multidisciplinary team, including the:

- doctor: diabetologist or general practitioner
- nurse: vascular, diabetes specialist or community
- vascular laboratory technician
- interventional radiologist
- vascular surgeon
- orthotist.

Peripheral vascular disease is usually only one manifestation of severe vascular disease throughout the body. Patients, often elderly, are extremely frail, with multisystem disease, including cardiovascular and cerebrovascular disease.

It may be the podiatrist who first encounters the severely dysvascular foot in diabetes, and an important aspect of the podiatrist's role is to alert other members of the healthcare team to the problem and ensure that rapid and appropriate care is delivered.

BACKGROUND TO ISCHAEMIA IN THE DIABETIC FOOT

Peripheral vascular disease in people with diabetes is usually bilateral, affecting both legs; multisegmental, involving more than one segment of the arteries involved; and distal, being located further down the leg than is usual in non-diabetic patients. In non-diabetics, iliac and femoral narrowing (stenosis) and blockages are more common, but in the diabetic patient stenosis and blockage often occur around the trifurcation of the tibial vessels at popliteal level (Fig. 6.1).

The joke is sometimes made that in non-diabetics the distribution of peripheral vascular disease runs from the nose down to the toes, whereas in diabetics it runs from the toes up to the nose.

The distal distribution of disease seen in diabetics is also seen in very elderly non-diabetic patients. The further down the leg the blockage or stenosis is, the less amenable it is to treatment because the vessel is smaller in diameter and more liable to be calcified. Examination of amputation or post-mortem specimens reveals that calcification in the medial wall of diabetic arteries is common. Vascular calcification can frequently be seen on X-ray (Fig. 6.2). The presence of calcification makes bypass surgery more difficult because it is hard to cut or clamp a calcified artery, and the surgeon's needle cannot easily penetrate the calcified arterial wall.

The youngest patient with severe peripheral vascular disease seen by the author was an 18-year-old girl, diabetic since the age of seven, with end-stage renal failure treated by haemodialysis and an acutely painful ischaemic left hallux, which improved after an angioplasty.

THE NATURAL HISTORY OF ISCHAEMIA IN THE DIABETIC FOOT

Peripheral vascular disease in non-diabetic patients is staged using the Fontaine system, as follows:

- Stage 1: intermittent claudication (calf muscle pain after walking a certain distance)
- Stage 2: rest pain
- Stage 3: ulceration
- Stage 4: gangrene.

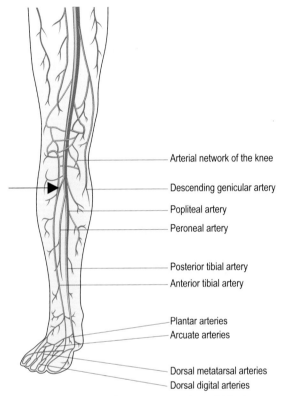

Arterial network of the knee

Descending genicular artery

Popliteal artery

Peroneal artery

Posterior tibial artery

Anterior tibial artery

Plantar arteries

Arcuate arteries

Dorsal metatarsal arteries

Dorsal digital arteries

Fig. 6.1   The arteries of the leg. Common sites of blockage and stenosis (arrowed) are at the trifurcation of the tibial vessels, just below the knee.

However, the Fontaine system is not useful for diabetic neuro-ischaemic patients because the presence of neuropathy and the distal nature of the vascular disease mean that many patients do not develop intermittent claudication or complain of rest pain. For many diabetic neuroischaemic patients, the first awareness that something is wrong comes with the development of ulcer or gangrene.

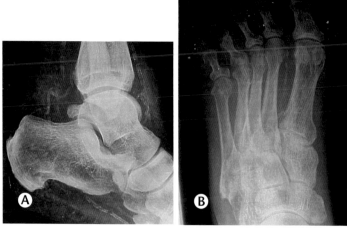

Fig. 6.2 In these X-rays of a diabetic neuroischaemic foot, vascular calcification is clearly seen (A) at the ankle and (B) in the space between the first metatarsal and the second metatarsal.

DEVELOPMENT OF ISCHAEMIA

Blood flow to the diabetic foot usually diminishes slowly and insidiously. Serial measurements show a gradual fall in the pressure index, and the Doppler signal changes from a healthy triphasic sound to a damped biphasic and then a monophasic or absent signal. If there is heavy calcification, the artery cannot be compressed and the pressure index remains high, so the examiner should, in addition to measuring the pressure index, listen to the signal and search for clinical signs of ischaemia.

Once the pressure index is below 0.7, healing of traumatic wounds or ulcers is seriously impaired and the ability to combat infection in the foot is diminished. There are signs of ischaemia, including hair loss, and thin, atrophic, shiny skin. (However, patients with neuropathy also often have hair loss within the distribution of their neuropathy.) Poorly perfused feet are usually cool, although if infected they can be deceptively warm. Symptoms of ischaemia are often absent.

Below a pressure index of 0.5, healing will be very protracted and may not occur at all, particularly when the patient has no symptoms and continues to walk. However, many very ischaemic feet do well so long as the skin is intact, and it is not until an injury occurs, when the foot is no longer able to mount the inflammatory response sufficient to achieve healing or fight infection, that ulcers develop and fail to heal. The level of blood flow required to sustain an intact foot is far lower that that which is required to heal an injured foot.

As the foot becomes seriously ischaemic, the colour of the skin gradually changes and becomes a deceptively healthy cherry pink colour, because capillaries dilate in an attempt to maximize perfusion of the tissues. However, the foot is very cold, (unless, as already stated, in addition to being ischaemic it is infected when it is sometimes warm). The cold, pink, painful ischaemic foot is sometimes called the sunset foot (Fig. 6.3).

However, feet with chronic ischaemia cover a wide spectrum, from the foot with weak pulses through to the cold, pink, and pulseless sunset foot, and on to the foot with indolent marginated ulcers and patches of necrosis.

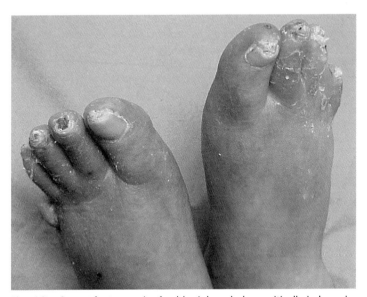

Fig. 6.3   Sunset feet – a pair of cold, pink, pulseless, critically ischaemic diabetic feet.

Some feet with chronic ischaemia are pale, with bluish or purple discoloration of the nail beds. The feet of patients with heart and lung disease may be blue or purple because of poor oxygenation of the blood from the central defect: in these circumstances the pedal pulses will be palpable unless there is also peripheral vascular disease.

Ischaemic feet may or may not be painful. Pain will depend on the degree of concurrent neuropathy and the location of the vascular disease, as already stated, and many patients have no symptoms of claudication or rest pain because the distal location of the vascular disease means that the affected area is within the distribution of their neuropathy.

Non-diabetic patients with peripheral vascular disease are usually aware that something is wrong: intermittent claudication limits walking and they take great care to avoid injuring their painful or sensitive ischaemic feet. Severe claudication and rest pain will result in a patient who walks very little. However, many people with diabetes and severe neuroischaemia are unaware that they have a problem with the circulation to their feet. They continue to walk freely and lack of protective pain sensation makes it likely that they will injure their delicate ischaemic tissues. The more they walk, the more likely they are to injure their feet. People with diabetes and neuroischaemic feet will therefore usually get into trouble sooner than non-diabetics with equally ischaemic feet and develop ulcers even when they have a higher pressure index than non-diabetic counterparts with no ulcers.

Non-diabetic patients with ischaemia who are aware that they have a problem and go to great lengths to prevent injury to their extremely sensitive feet will often do well until their pressure index has fallen to 0.3 or lower. This might be why people with ischaemia and concurrent neuropathy tend to develop problems with their feet earlier than people without neuropathy. Furthermore, many people with peripheral vascular disease and diabetes also have eye problems, including diabetic retinopathy and/or cataract, and cannot see their feet clearly enough to inspect them for colour change or breaks in the skin.

Even if ischaemic patients also have severe neuropathy and sites of high pressure on the plantar surface of the foot, they do not develop exuberant callus. When blood flow diminishes there seems to be a reduction in callus formation. A small study at King's College Hospital investigated callus formation around both neuropathic and ischaemic ulcers in diabetic patients and found that few ischaemic ulcers were associated with callus. For this reason, unless there has been an incident of direct trauma causing injury to the foot, such as treading on a sharp object or pulling a piece of loose skin off the foot, plantar ulceration is rare in the neuroischaemic foot. Instead, it is the margins of the foot, including the tips of the toes, that are the most common sites of ulceration.

The factor that triggers an ischaemic ulcer is often oedema, which renders the shoes too tight and results in areas of pressure on the margins of the foot. The patient does not perceive the problem because of concurrent neuropathy. Oedema is common in diabetic patients with peripheral vascular disease, and is usually due to concurrent cardiac and/or renal problems. Sub-ungual ulceration, beneath a thickened toenail, is also commonly seen in the neuroischaemic diabetic foot.

It may be true that neuroischaemic tissues are much more vulnerable to injury than tissues with normal vasculature and innervation. In particular, patients with end-stage renal failure and peripheral vascular disease seem to be particularly vulnerable to severe damage from an apparently small insult (Fig. 6.4).

■ Aims of management of chronic ischaemia

The aims of management of the neuroischaemic foot are:

- To protect the foot from injury by providing education and regular preventive foot care from an experienced podiatrist, and by treating oedema, cardiac and renal problems, hypertension and hyperlipidaemia. Many patients will be on aspirin and statins.
- To encourage the patient not to use tobacco products.
- To provide suitable shoes to protect the vulnerable margins of the foot.
- To monitor the vascular status and to explore the possibility of vascular intervention if the pressure index falls below 0.5, intermittent claudication or rest pain develop, or the patient develops ulcers, infection or gangrene.
- To offer follow-up care within a multidisciplinary diabetic foot clinic for all patients with severe ischaemia.

Self-care is wholly inappropriate for the neuroischaemic foot, and patients, their relatives, and other healthcare professionals should not be asked to cut the nails unless a podiatry service is not available, in which circumstances the nails should be filed in one direction, very carefully, gently and frequently, to control their length and thickness.

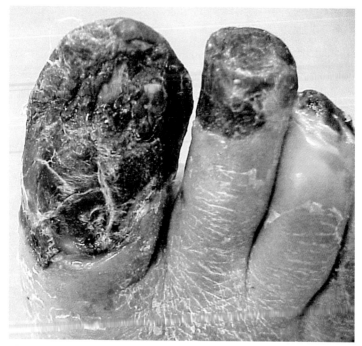

Fig. 6.4 This patient in end-stage renal failure developed necrosis after his second toe was pricked to obtain a capillary blood sample.

ACUTE ISCHAEMIA

Legs become acutely ischaemic when a major vessel blocks off. This can occur suddenly, without any history of previous vascular problems, or as an acute event superimposed on a background of chronic ischaemia.

Acute ischaemia is a clinical emergency requiring very rapid treatment if the leg (and often the patient's life) is to be saved. The patient presents with coldness, pain or paraesthesiae (tingling, pins and needles) and bluish-grey or purplish mottling and pallor of the distal part of the leg, of recent onset (Fig 6.5). The pedal pulses are impalpable, and sometimes great weakness and even paralysis of the

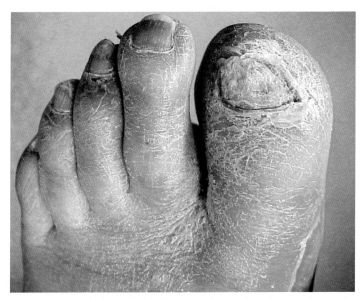

Fig. 6.5   Acute ischaemia. No flow was detected on Dopplering and the transcutaneous oxygen measurement was 5. The foot and lower leg were icy cold, with bluish mottling. The patient was admitted to hospital immediately and underwent distal bypass the next day, and the foot was saved.

affected limb is present. There is a dramatic temperature gradient, where the distal area of the limb suddenly becomes icy cold below the site of arterial blockage.

If the neuropathy is profound, the patient might not feel severe pain but will usually still be aware that there is a problem with the foot.

■ Rapid action

This is a clinical emergency. The patient should be taken immediately to the nearest hospital where a vascular team (with interventional radiologist and vascular surgeon) is available to assess him immediately and take steps to unblock or bypass the affected vessel. Procedures that may be attempted include:

- bypass
- angioplasty
- embolectomy.

It may be possible to dissolve the blood clot which is blocking the vessel by using a clot-busting drug such as streptokinase.

Bypass

This is a major operation with not insignificant morbidity and mortality and is not undertaken lightly. It takes several hours to perform. Common sites of bypass include:

- iliofemoral
- femoropopliteal
- femorodistal.

The most successful grafts are of autologous vein (from the patient's own leg). Synthetic grafts are available but their survival is greatly reduced compared with autologous grafts. Many patients with peripheral vascular disease also have disease of the coronary arteries, and leg veins have frequently already been used for a coronary artery bypass graft (CABG) by the time the patient develops significant peripheral vascular disease. In these circumstances many surgeons prefer to harvest veins from the patient's arms rather than use a synthetic graft.

During the perioperative period, good control of diabetes, usually with insulin, is mandatory.

Post-bypass management

The foot should be checked every day to ensure that pulses can still be palpated in the pedal arteries. An inspection of the foot is also made searching for ischaemic areas, which may first present as bluish areas that initially look like bruising but subsequently become necrotic. It is difficult to assess the true extent or depth of necrosis before several days have passed and the necrosis has demarcated.

Post-bypass feet with extensive areas of full thickness necrosis can sometimes be saved with careful follow up in a multidisciplinary foot clinic. It is very important to offload the heels on the operating table and during the perioperative period to prevent necrosis.

Care of leg wounds post-bypass

Leg wounds that lie over the new graft, and also the area where the vein has been harvested, should be checked regularly for cellulitis, purulent discharge, or necrosis. Infection and dehiscence of the wounds are not uncommon. Ideally, patients will be followed up regularly in a joint clinic by the vascular surgeon, diabetic physician, nurse, orthotist, and podiatrist. Heaped up necrosis, slough, and crusted exudates can be debrided away together with what is clearly non-viable tissue: however, it should never be forgotten that beneath the eschar is the new graft and that if this is damaged or becomes infected then the leg is at great risk of amputation. Furthermore, a failed leg bypass generally necessitates an above-knee amputation and often leads to the death of the patient.

Postoperative oedema and discoloration

After a bypass, most patients develop oedema of the operated limb, which usually persists. Some develop brownish discoloration around the foot and ankle (in the Afro Caribbean foot this manifests itself as a darker area), which might be due to post-inflammatory hyper-pigmentation and usually persists.

▓ Aims of management of acute ischaemia

- To quantitate the degree of ischaemia.
- To admit the patient for urgent vascular intervention: angioplasty or bypass.
- To provide follow-up care in a specialist multidisciplinary diabetic foot clinic.

Acute ischaemia of sudden onset is quite rare. Chronic ischaemia, which gradually deteriorates until the ischaemia is critical, is the more common presentation.

CHRONIC ISCHAEMIA

From work conducted at King's College Hospital, we have found that around 75% of ischaemic diabetic patients with ulceration respond well to conservative care from a multidisciplinary diabetic foot team so long as ulcers are caught early and treatment is not delayed. However, a quarter of patients will benefit from vascular interventions such as angioplasty or distal bypass. If these treatments are not available then it is inevitable that some diabetic patients with neuro-ischaemic feet will come, in the end, to major amputation. Many neuroischaemic patients will first die from stroke or myocardial infarction, as most patients with peripheral vascular disease also have cardiovascular and cerebrovascular disease.

■ The joint vascular diabetic foot clinic

At King's, we organize a weekly joint vascular clinic with the vascular surgeon and his team. Patients with indolent ischaemic ulcers or gangrene have duplex scans and transcutaneous oxymetry levels performed and are then seen in the outpatient diabetic foot clinic by the vascular team. If vascular intervention is deemed necessary, there is a fast-track system for performing angiography and angioplasty, often in the day-surgery unit. Patients who undergo a procedure are followed-up in the joint vascular clinic and, if they deteriorate, they can thus be seen and assessed by the full team very quickly.

PREVENTIVE FOOT CARE FOR THE DYSVASCULAR DIABETIC FOOT

■ Care of nails

Only experienced, fully trained, HPC registered podiatrists should be expected to cut the toenails of patients with severe peripheral vascular disease; in these circumstances relatives and nurses should never be asked to provide nail care. Nails should be cut straight across, not so short that the seal between nail bed and nail plate is broken, and not left so long that they can catch on socks (Fig 6.6).

If nails are thickened or gryphotic, the thickness of the nail should be very carefully reduced either by gentle filing or by shaving off layers of nail with a scalpel in thin slickets, as otherwise pressure from the thickened nail can lead to ischaemic ulceration of the nail bed. It is essential not to break the skin but it should also be remembered that neglected nails will eventually always cause problems. When cutting the nails, a very careful nibbling approach should be adopted, as cutting the entire nail in one piece can often cause it to split and damage the nail bed.

Nail sulci, the grooves of soft tissue at the sides of the nail into which the nail fits, should be very gently cleared of debris and the edge of the nail plate filed smooth with a Blacks file, taking great

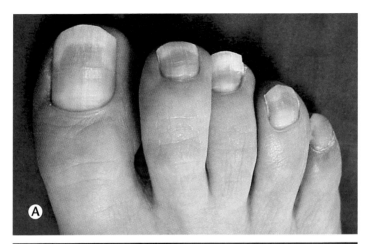

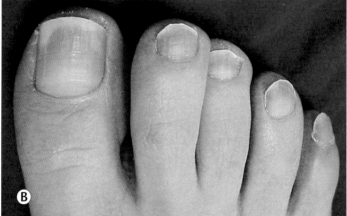

Fig. 6.6   (A) A critically ischaemic foot where no vascular intervention is possible. The pressure index is 0.3. Note the purplish colour of the nail beds. The nails need to be cut with great care to avoid injuring ischaemic tissues. (B) The nails have been carefully cut and filed, and the patient will be seen at monthly intervals for preventive foot care.

care not to damage the tissues of the sulcus. Some practitioners like to soften any debris around the nail (onychophosis) with a few drops of topically applied hydrogen peroxide.

If the nail plate is pressing on the sulcus, or if a splinter of nail has penetrated the sulcus, and the problem cannot be cleared with the Black's file, it may be possible to remove a small sliver of nail with a scalpel without causing trauma to the surrounding soft tissues.

When working with nails on seriously ischaemic feet, the practitioner needs always to mentally balance the dangers of operating, and possibly causing irritation, inflammation and tissue breakdown, against the dangers of leaving the sulcus loaded with debris, or with the nail edge causing pressure on the sulcus, which can also lead to irritation, inflammation and tissue breakdown.

If there is real dilemma, it should be discussed with the patient and his family, and other members of the healthcare team, who should always be involved in difficult decisions. If this is not done, there is a danger that the podiatrist will be blamed if problems develop after treatment. (see Chapter 9).

■ Corns and calluses on neuroischaemic feet

This subject is discussed in further detail in Chapters 1 and 8. Although callus and corns are rare in the neuroischaemic foot, when they are present their management is particularly challenging. Plaques of callus are thin, hard, and glassy in consistency, and it is difficult to remove them without causing injury. The scalpel blade is very likely to slip and it is not easy to assess the depth of the callus from its texture, which is uniformly hard and glassy. It is the author's impression that some patients, and in particular, Afro-Caribbean patients, are prone to develop corns and calluses even in the presence of severe ischaemia and these need to be removed with great care. Podiatrists are usually taught that every scrap of corn and callus should be removed from the foot. However, if the foot is neuroischaemic then it is better to under-operate and see the patient at more frequent intervals than to risk damaging ischaemic tissues. In these circumstances it should be accepted that it is sometimes impossible to clear away every scrap of corn and callus.

■ Care of dry skin

Excessively thick areas of dry hyperkeratosis should be carefully debrided with a scalpel, following which the patient is asked to apply an emollient twice a day. E45® cream usually works well. Difficult cases may benefit from a urea-containing cream such as Calmurid®.

■ Care of skin flaps and flakes

Many patients find it difficult to resist pulling and picking at loose flakes of dry skin. Regular application of an emollient and use of a scalpel by the podiatrist to debride edges of callus that stand free or proud of the surrounding skin are helpful. Patients with a habit of picking at their feet can be advised always to keep their feet covered with cotton socks except when they are in the bath or shower.

METABOLIC CONTROL FOR THE VASCULAR PATIENT

■ Hyperlipidaemia

Good management of hyperlipidaemia (and hypertrigliceridaemia) are essential for diabetic patients at risk of vascular disease or with current vascular disease. Patients should receive dietary advice to reduce fat intake and appropriate drugs, including statins and aspirin. The Hope Study is the evidence base for this (for further details see Chapter 2).

■ Weight loss

It is easy to instruct patients to lose weight but many patients find it impossible to succeed. Some patients have been offered barosurgery, where an inflatable device is inserted into the stomach so that it is impossible for the patient to overeat. However, in patients with neuropathy affecting the gastrointestinal tract the results of baro-surgery can be very disappointing.

■ Smoking

It is essential for neuroischaemic patients to stop smoking. This is easy to say but difficult to achieve. Tobacco is a strongly addictive drug and it is very hard for patients to give it up. Unequivocal advice should be given, together with information about local smoking cessation programmes and sympathetic support. Many elderly unwell smokers say that tobacco is one of the few pleasures left to them. One of the author's patients, who had undergone a below-knee amputation for peripheral vascular disease, announced that he had had no problems giving up smoking. However, on his next visit he was observed to be taking snuff in the waiting area. Another patient commented on the efficacy of nicotine patches – he was wearing eight of them at the same time!

EDUCATIONAL CONTROL FOR THE VASCULAR PATIENT

Special education should be provided for neuroischaemic patients, with particular emphasis on the need to wear suitable shoes, to avoid trauma from walking barefooted, and never to apply direct heat or ice packs to the feet. Patients should be warned that if their feet feel cold, the only safe treatment is to wear warm socks, and that electric blankets and hot water bottles or other methods of directly applying heat to the feet are very dangerous when the blood supply is poor.

MECHANICAL CONTROL FOR VASCULAR PATIENTS

Many neuroischaemic patients are old and frail and do not go out much. Their main desire is for lightweight shoes that are suitable for wearing round the house and that are easy to put on, take off, fasten, and unfasten. Many such patients are reluctant to wear bespoke shoes on the grounds that they are too heavy. For patients who find it difficult to reach their feet there are donning and doffing aids. Elastic laces may be useful and velcro fastenings are easier than laces. In the United Kingdom, many people like to have house shoes as well as going-out shoes.

Patients with high-risk neuroischaemic feet should have all shoe purchases vetted by the podiatrist. Reputable shoe shops and mail-order companies will provide shoes on a sale or return basis if it is explained that the patient has special needs, so long as the shoes have not been worn. Patients and their families should receive advice on the size and style of shoes and patients with deformity or oedema may need bespoke shoes from the orthotist. Shoes should be extra depth and wide fitting, with cushioned insoles, and any significant deformity should be accommodated within bespoke footwear. Patients should not go barefoot, nor wear slippers around the house except for the short walk to and from the bathroom at the beginning and end of the day and for any additional nocturnal trips.

■ Common problems are caused by

- Deliberate or inadvertent application of excessive heat or cold: hot water bottles, electric blankets or heating pads with faulty

thermostats, overly hot temperature of baths and showers (above 45°C is dangerous), standing in the snow, leaking shoes.
- Open-toed or flimsy shoes: some patients with sensitive feet like to wear sandals, which do not protect the feet sufficiently from external trauma or foreign bodies.
- Dropping objects on feet.
- Foot spas.
- Worn or rough places or prominent seams in shoes.
- Walking barefoot.
- Trying to cut own toe nails.
- Lumpy darns or holes in socks or stockings.
- Ill-fitting shoes or socks.
- Foreign bodies in shoes.
- Sharp objects penetrating thin-soled shoes or slippers.

All of these problems can be eliminated if great care is taken to protect the foot and if patients and carers think ahead with imagination. However, when concurrent neuropathy is present the patient may not perceive the risk or the need to protect the feet, and if the patient has visual problems and cannot see clearly it is difficult to detect problems. In these circumstances, the protective role of family and carers is of tremendous importance, and frequent appointments with the footcare team can greatly improve outcomes for vulnerable patients.

EMERGENCY SERVICES

If pain, colour change or ulceration develops, then a diabetic patient should be seen by a specialist team within 24 h (Fig. 6.7). This is now laid down in the National Institute of Clinical Excellence (NICE) guidelines for the management of the diabetic foot, and accommodation of this requirement should be planned for and built into all podiatry programmes. In practice, it may be difficult to achieve this if the patient is elderly, frail, or socially isolated; and a precise definition of what is meant by 'specialist' is not given in the guidelines. It is essential for hospital and community podiatrists to work together and arrange an urgent home visit, if necessary, and equally important that the patient is not seen in isolation by a solitary podiatrist who has no access to other members of the multidisciplinary team.

Vascular management programmes for each stage are described below:

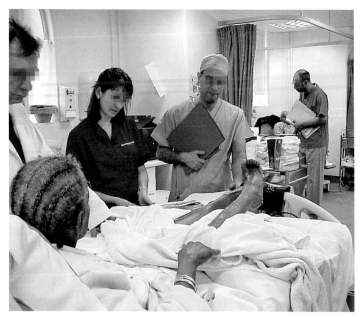

Fig. 6.7 Neuroischaemic patients with gangrene should be managed by a multidisciplinary team. Here, a patient is seen by the physician, the diabetic foot practitioner and the vascular surgeon.

CARE PLANS FOR VASCULAR PATIENTS

■ The Stage 1 normal diabetic foot

Annual review. Checking pulses. Visual inspection for signs of ischaemia (atrophic skin, etc.).

■ The Stage 2 intact neuroischaemic foot

Quantitate ischaemia with one or more of the following methods:

● pulse palpation
● Doppler
● transcutaneous pO_2.

Offer routine preventive foot care at sufficiently frequent intervals. Assess footwear. Teach patients they are at risk of ulceration and gangrene and that there is a need for regular inspection of the feet for:

- colour change
- swelling
- pain or throbbing
- breaks in the skin.

Many patients with neuroischaemia are elderly and frail. In addition to peripheral vascular disease they often have concurrent cardiac and cerebrovascular problems. Many of them are incapable of looking after their feet, inspecting them and detecting problems early, and it is essential for family, friends or healthcare professionals to rally round and help to develop a programme of care which will keep them safe.

■ The Stage 3 ulcerated neuroischaemic foot

Preventive foot care as described for Stage 2 above is important for Stage 3 patients, and in addition they need expert care of their ulcers, preferably in a hospital-based multidisciplinary foot clinic (for further details of debridement and wound care for Stage 3 neuroischaemic feet, see Chapter 8).

Neuroischaemic diabetic feet with ulceration are at great risk of developing infection and necrosis. If blood flow is poor, then the vascular component of the inflammatory response is defective. This means that wounds cannot heal quickly and that patients cannot fight infection well (Fig. 6.8). Signs and symptoms of infection are frequently diminished. Stage 3 neuroischaemic feet need to be inspected regularly.

Dressing the Stage 3 foot

Most hospital foot clinics work together with the community district nursing service to ensure that patients with high-risk feet are seen regularly and that ulcers are frequently redressed. When the patient is old and frail and incapable of self-care, and cannot feel pain or see the feet clearly, a daily visit from the community nurse is best practice. The common belief that wounds that are redressed very frequently may be disturbed, with impairment of the healing process, is dangerous if applied to the insensitive neuroischaemic diabetic foot, where the danger of failing to detect deterioration is greater than the danger of disturbing the wound.

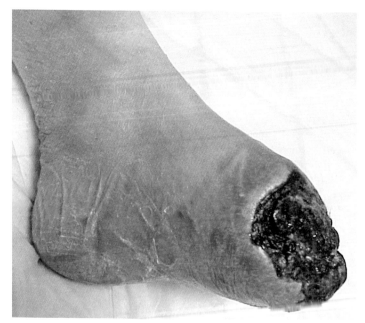

Fig 6.8 This neuroischaemic patient underwent a transmetatarsal amputation and the severely ischaemic surgical wound became necrotic.

Care should be taken when choosing and applying dressings to neuroischaemic feet. Moist wound care can lead to maceration of slough and necrosis, which is then an ideal growth medium for microorganisms, and also renders the wound harder to assess. This is also a problem if gels or chemical debriding agents are used. Use of too much tape risks tearing the skin: the author has found this to be a particular problem with Micropore® tape. Encircling the toe or foot with tight bandage or tape risks a dangerous reduction in blood flow. It should be remembered that oedema may be fluctuant and that a loosely applied bandage will become too tight if the foot swells. Blue-line tubular bandage is a very useful dressing holder, and it is unfortunate that it is so expensive that many centres cannot afford to use it.

The use of undiluted antiseptics or caustics is always contraindicated for the diabetic neuroischaemic foot.

Pain in the Stage 3 neuroischaemic foot
In the absence of infection, pain is usually due to ischaemia and the ulcerated patient who develops new or increased pain should be reviewed urgently by the vascular team.

▦ The Stage 4 infected neuroischaemic foot
It is difficult for the dysvascular foot to fight infection. It has been our policy at King's to prescribe systemic antibiotics early if patients are severely ischaemic or have a previous history of severe infection.

It is sometimes said that there is no point in prescribing antibiotics to patients with ischaemia because the blood supply will be too poor for them to reach the foot. However, unless the foot is entirely gangrenous, there will be sufficient blood flow to transport useful amounts of antibiotics to viable tissue and antibiotics will diffuse across from viable tissue into adjoining necrotic tissues. This was demonstrated by an interesting study from Eastern Europe of patients who underwent major amputation because of gangrene. Patients were given antibiotics the day before surgery and, after the ischaemic limb was amputated, levels of antibiotics in the tissues were measured. Ischaemia should not be used as an excuse for failure to treat infection.

There is a dilemma to be faced in patients with severe ischaemia who present with serious infection, sometimes associated with wet gangrene, a collection of pus, or sloughy liquefied tissue. There is an urgent need for debridement but the circulation may not be sufficient to heal the resulting surgical wound. Attempts should be made to improve the circulation by vascular intervention in this situation, but where vascular intervention is impossible, the foot should be surgically debrided to drain obviously necrotic wet infected material and drain pus and a trial of conservative care undertaken. Some ischaemic feet respond surprisingly well once infection is controlled. However, revascularization should be regarded as an essential component of infection management in the critically ischaemic and infected neuroischaemic diabetic foot.

Pain in the Stage 4 neuroischaemic foot
Severe pain in the neuroischaemic foot may be due to infection, and is often relieved by treatment with antibiotics. However, pain may

also be due to increasing ischaemia. As already stated, any patient with new pain or increasing pain in an ischaemic foot needs specialist assessment without delay.

■ The Stage 5 necrotic neuroischaemic foot

At one time, gangrene in the neuroischaemic foot was regarded as the end of the road and patients with gangrene were offered above-knee amputations. It is now realized that there is a place for conservative care even in diabetic patients with gangrene in poorly perfused feet that have had unsuccessful revascularization or where angioplasty or bypass were not feasible. The programme of conservative care is as follows:

- Pain relief: if the feet are painful, the patient is given liberal analgesia.
- Reduction of oedema with appropriate drugs.
- Optimal control of diabetes. Most patients are put on insulin.
- Preventive foot care for nails and skin.
- Gentle podiatric debridement of ulcers and gangrene (see Chapter 8) at intervals of no more than 2 weeks.
- Sterile, non-adherent dressings, held in place by light bandaging: gangrenous toes are separated by an interdigital dry dressing.
- Extra-depth, wide-fitting shoes, to protect ulcers and the vulnerable margins of the foot and to accommodate dressings.
- Rest and elevation.
- Prevention and control of infection. Frequent monitoring with swabs or tissue samples: antibiotics as appropriate.
- Careful education of patient and family so that they understand the signs and symptoms of deterioration and will report them rapidly and seek same day help if they arise.

Some patients refuse major amputation and their wishes must always be respected (Fig. 6.9).

■ The Stage 6 neuroischaemic major amputee

The diabetic patient who has already lost one foot due to peripheral vascular disease is among the most high-risk patients the podiatrist is likely to encounter. In most cases, rehabilitation is not very successful and patients often become wheelchair users. Despite this, the remaining foot and leg are exceedingly precious because patients with one leg

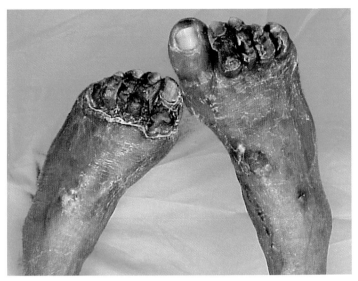

Fig. 6.9 This neuroischaemic patient presented late, with wet gangrene, and no vascular intervention was possible. She refused a major amputation and was managed conservatively. She was given bilateral Scotchcast boots, the demarcation line between gangrene and viable tissue was debrided every week by the podiatrist, and the physician prescribed antibiotics. The necrosis became dry and well demarcated and she was able to go home. She was offered regular follow-up appointments in the joint vascular/diabetic foot clinic.

are usually able to transfer from wheelchair to lavatory and to bed, and thus retain some independence.

The perioperative time is fraught with danger for neuroischaemic diabetic major amputees. They are at risk of developing pressure ulcers on the trolley in casualty while they wait for a bed, on the operating table when their leg is amputated, and in bed during the recovery period. While being rehabilitated, they risk falls and trauma to the remaining foot. It is essential for podiatrists to work together with the physiotherapists and other members of the rehabilitation team, to minimize the risk of trauma and observe the remaining foot carefully so that problems can be detected early.

Case study

An 82-year-old woman with type 2 diabetes had suffered a stroke at the age of 74. She was wheelchair bound and lived with her daughter. She was admitted to another hospital after inhaling milk and developing aspiration pneumonia, while in hospital she developed bilateral necrosis of both heels.

She was discharged to the care of the district nursing service and referred to King's as an emergency when rapidly spreading wet gangrene threatened to destroy her entire left foot. Associated pain was very severe. She was admitted for pain control, vascular assessment, and intravenous antibiotics. No vascular intervention was possible and, because of the extent of the necrosis, she was offered a below-knee amputation. However, she communicated very firmly that she would rather die than have an amputation and was managed conservatively. Once the necrosis was dry and fairly well demarcated, she was discharged home to her daughter and came to the clinic at weekly intervals for debridement. Three months later she suffered a fatal stroke at home. Her daughter said she was very glad that her mother had not undergone amputation and had died peacefully at home.

At King's we have provided a special podiatry service for major amputees attending the local orthotics and prosthetics centre.

Programmes of care for diabetic major amputees will depend on the stage of the remaining foot. However, it is also important for podiatrists to be aware that diabetic major amputees are at risk of developing problems with the stump, which may become neuropathic, ischaemic, or infected.

A literature search reveals alarming mortality and morbidity among diabetic major amputees, with one half dying within 3 years of the amputation, and half of the survivors losing the contralateral limb. However, a retrospective study of 38 patients with diabetes, who had undergone major amputation and subsequently been referred to King's diabetic foot clinic for follow-up care, over a mean period of over 4 years, found that although 26 patients developed foot ulcers and several needed angioplasty or bypass, only two patients needed major amputation of the remaining leg. All these patients were cared for by a multidisciplinary team of podiatrist, nurse, physician, orthotist, interventional radiologist, and vascular surgeon.

■ The end-stage renal failure foot with neuroischaemia

Many patients with end-stage renal failure develop severe peripheral vascular disease, which is often difficult to treat because of widespread vascular calcification. Even in the absence of peripheral vascular disease, the renal foot has a remarkable propensity to develop extensive gangrene from a tiny, apparently minor, injury. The reasons for this are not entirely clear, but because of this great care must be taken when debriding ulcers and gangrene on renal feet, because of the risk of causing die back, with rapid proximal advance of necrosis.

Patients on haemodialysis are treated with blood-thinning agents and should be debrided with caution for 24 h after dialysing. Some renal patients have such a long history of serious illness with dramatic features that it can be difficult for them to prioritize their foot care sufficiently. Traumatic foot injuries are particularly common, and it may be that the tissues of the renal foot are more susceptible to injury than the tissues of patients without renal disease.

■ Podiatric assessment and management of end-stage renal failure patients treated with renal transplantation

Between 1987 and 1991 the author followed 50 patients with diabetes and end-stage renal failure treated by renal transplantation to try to elucidate the reasons why morbidity and mortality are so high among diabetic patients with end-stage renal failure. Until then it had been postulated that the reason was severe peripheral vascular disease. All patients in the study group underwent screening for the presence of neuropathy and ischaemia and a history was taken of previous foot problems. Feet were checked at every monthly visit to the renal unit, patients were offered regular podiatry, and all foot-related lesions, investigative and interventional procedures, and outcomes were recorded. Only 12 patients had absent pulses and a pressure index below 1, indicating ischaemia. Only two patients underwent major amputation during the period of the study, both of whom had ischaemia. There was a reduction in gangrene and major amputations among study patients compared to a similar group of diabetic renal patients studied during the 4 years previous to the study, who had not received regular podiatry.

MANAGEMENT OF GANGRENE IN THE NEUROISCHAEMIC FOOT

Gangrene in the diabetic neuroischaemic foot is difficult to manage. The team has two options. The first is surgical removal of the gangrenous part. The second is a conservative approach.

If surgery is to be considered then it is important to optimize perfusion of the foot with angioplasty or bypass first, if feasible. If these procedures cannot be undertaken, then surgery should be performed only if it is essential and is the only means of preventing the spread of infection, or because pain in the area adjoining the gangrene is excruciating and unremitting and does not respond to analgesia. It is always unfortunate when patients are subjected to salami procedures, where one operation after another is performed, none heals, and the foot and leg are gradually whittled away. It is important, preoperatively, to measure oxygen tension in the skin to determine whether surgical wounds have a chance of healing.

■ Conservative care of gangrenous toes

The conservative approach to gangrene is described in Chapter 8. Many gangrenous feet will heal given meticulous care with special emphasis on preventing and controlling infection.

In a small retrospective study conducted by the author of 21 patients with full-thickness gangrene of a toe in a diabetic neuroischaemic foot and in whom vascular intervention was not possible, 17 patients healed with conservative care, which culminated in successful autoamputation of the gangrenous digit leaving a healed stump. Only four patients came to a major amputation.

The foot sometimes benefits from removal of a necrotic toe by the podiatrist, if the necrotic toe is causing problems due to contact with adjoining toes, or retraction. Removal of the toe enables the podiatrist to debulk necrotic material from the demarcation line between gangrene and viable tissue (Fig 6.10).

It should not be forgotten that gangrene in the neuroischaemic diabetic foot is not necessarily the result of ischaemia and may be due to infection, and that the signs and symptoms of infection are diminished in the neuroischaemic foot. Pain in the ischaemic foot is also often caused by infection. The author has seen many diabetic patients, referred for a second opinion as to whether amputation was inevitable, in great pain from their gangrenous feet, who responded

Fig. 6.10 (A) This man developed necrosis of the hallux following an episode of infection. His foot was too ischaemic for the toe to be amputated as with a pressure index of 0.4 the wound was unlikely to heal and it was not feasible to improve blood flow to the toe with a vascular procedure. The dried, mummified toe has retracted over the neighbouring toe to such an extent that when he walks the second toe is traumatized and a patch of superficial necrosis is developing on the dorsum of the second toe. (B) The proximal portion of the toe has been amputated through the interphalangeal joint by the podiatrist. The area of the toe which was causing problems to its neighbour has thus been removed. No injury has been caused to viable tissue. It will now be possible to debride necrotic material from the demarcation line between gangrene and viable tissue. The foot healed in 3 months.

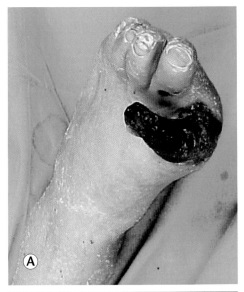

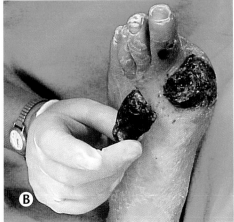

very well to systemic antibiotics, and healed after being offered multidisciplinary care even though vascular intervention was not feasible.

■ Balancing the dangers of operating or of not operating on the neuroischaemic foot

To amputate or not to amputate can be a contentious issue and podiatrists should be familiar with arguments commonly used for and against amputation.

Dangers of operating

- Amputations and surgical wounds may never heal. There may then be a need for further surgical procedures, which in their turn may not heal, which is painful and distressing for patient and family.
- Morbidity and mortality are high in elderly, frail patients.
- Distal bypass is a major operation.
- Angiography dye may further damage kidneys in patients with renal impairment and lead to end-stage renal failure.
- When patients have a short lifespan they should not spend a large proportion of it in hospital recovering from surgery.
- Surgery leaves large wounds, which may never heal, or healing may be very protracted.
- In the early stages of gangrene it can be difficult to assess which tissue is viable and surgery may be unnecessarily extensive.
- Many patients admitted to hospital for surgery develop pressure ulcers.
- The cost of long-term hospital stays for diabetic foot patients is phenomenal.
- Infections with resistant microorganisms are common in diabetic foot patients who have undergone surgery.

Dangers of not operating

- Surgery may be the only way of relieving pain.
- The diabetic foot does not tolerate the presence of pus under pressure, slough or infected tissue. Severe infection may not resolve without drainage and removal of sloughy infected tissue and it is difficult to control severe infection without surgery.
- Infection can kill patients unless surgery is undertaken.

- Necrotizing fasciitis and gas gangrene can destroy the foot and leg with alarming rapidity and surgery is the only effective treatment.
- Unless gangrenous toes are amputated there is always a risk of infection supervening.
- Conservative care of autoamputating gangrenous toes takes many months.
- If patients are wheelchair or bed bound then amputation will not affect their mobility.

Advantages of major amputation

- Cures agonizing rest pain.
- Means that the patient no longer has to attend the hospital so frequently.
- No need for regular wound care.
- Lifesaving in cases of severe infection and acute ischaemia.
- Gets the patient home quickly.
- A good prosthesis is better than an indolent ulcerated foot or unstable Charcot joint.

Disadvantages of major amputation

- Within 3 years half of the patients will be dead.
- Within 3 years half of the survivors will have lost both legs.
- Successful rehabilitation is not the norm: the majority of patients will be wheelchair bound.
- Many patients will lose their independence and no longer be able to live alone at home.
- There is a high incidence of problems in the remaining foot. If a leg that is potentially salvageable is amputated and the remaining leg develops severe problems, the patient may end up with bilateral major amputations, unable even to transfer, and with very poor quality of life.
- The stump may develop ulcers.
- The stump wound may never heal.
- The remaining leg will be overloaded and prone to ulceration.

WORKING IN ISOLATION

The podiatrist who sees deterioration in a diabetic neuroischaemic foot but cannot persuade the GP to refer the patient to the vascular team faces a special dilemma. Sometimes, sending the patient directly to casualty may be the only solution: however, an inexperienced house officer in casualty may underestimate the situation. It is necessary to foster close links between the hospital diabetic foot clinic and the community podiatry service, so that patients can be seen and assessed quickly by experienced practitioners, preferably in a joint vascular clinic.

7 Non-ulcerative pathologies

Rest, rest, perturbed spirit …
The time is out of joint.

William Shakespeare, Hamlet IV. 182

The non-ulcerative diabetic foot pathologies include:

- Charcot's osteoarthropathy
- painful neuropathy
- pathological fractures.

CHARCOT'S OSTEOARTHROPATHY

This is a mysterious and unpredictable affliction of bone and joint in the neuropathic foot. Patients with combined sensory and autonomic neuropathy develop a progressive destructive osteoarthropathy. This can lead to severe deformity and/or instability of the affected joint, often associated with indolent ulceration. Although more than 40 different names are used to describe the condition, the most accurate term is Charcot's osteoarthropathy, for this disease affects both bone and joint and is associated with the name of Professor Jean Martin Charcot, by whom it was described in the 19th century. Charcot's patients had syphilis; diabetes is the most common associated condition in Europe in the 21st century.

■ Staging the Charcot foot

Many groups have attempted to describe distinct stages in the progression of this destructive arthropathy, but for practical purposes there are three stages as follows:

- active stage: acute onset and bony destruction – red, hot, swollen foot (Fig. 7.1)
- resolution stage: redness, warmth, and swelling settle but there might be residual deformity (Fig. 7.2)

Fig. 7.1 This red, hot, swollen, acute Charcot foot developed 2 days after the patient visited the diabetic foot clinic for removal of a total contact cast applied to heal an indolent neuropathic ulcer. He had been advised to rest the foot as much as possible but went shopping.

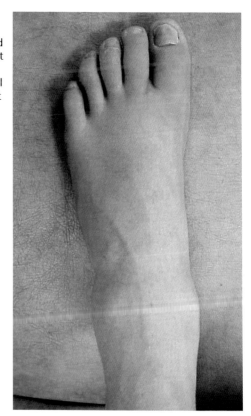

- rehabilitation phase: if this is conducted too speedily there is great danger of relapse.

Active stage of acute onset and bony destruction

Patients first present with redness, warmth, and swelling of a foot or part of a foot. The affected foot is at least 2°C hotter than the other foot and may be as much as 7 or 8° hotter. (A good blood supply is present: ischaemia usually protects patients from developing a Charcot foot.) The affected foot is always redder, warmer, and more swollen than the unaffected foot. The redness is usually duskier than the florid red of a staphylococcal cellulitis. The discoloration is diffuse.

Fig. 7.2 This patient was left with a severe medial convexity deformity of his Charcot foot.
When the problem first developed it was misdiagnosed as osteoarthritis and he was told that exercise would help.

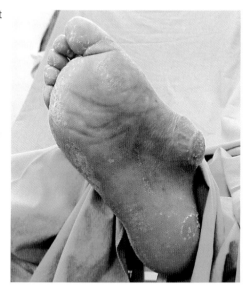

On questioning, the patient often remembers undergoing a trauma such as a trip, slip, twist, or fall, or a period of increased or unusual activity, like Christmas shopping, carrying heavy luggage, or walking on cobbled streets or uneven pavements. Other patients develop the condition after a surgical procedure, a period of immobility on bed rest, or after a below-knee cast has been removed and they have resumed walking.

Around 30% of acute Charcot patients report some degree of pain or discomfort in the affected foot but the degree of pain is always less than would be expected in a foot with normal protective pain sensation and a comparable injury.

The differential diagnosis includes cellulitis and gout. Charcot's osteoarthropathy can also be mistaken for osteomyelitis, septic arthritis, rheumatoid arthritis, osteoarthritis, and deep vein thrombosis. Any of the above can develop concurrently with an acute Charcot's osteoarthropathy and render correct diagnosis very challenging. It can also be very difficult to differentiate between Charcot's osteoarthropathy and a soft tissue injury such as a sprain, or a severe infection. A soft tissue injury will heal quicker than a Charcot and infection is unlikely if there is no ulcer or other portal of entry, but there can always be exceptions to these rules. Gout can be excluded by a blood test.

Charcot's osteoarthropathy is quite uncommon and is frequently misdiagnosed by inexperienced practitioners. Many healthcare professionals have either never seen it or have failed to recognize it. Some unfortunate patients with red, hot, swollen feet who consult inexperienced practitioners are told to 'walk more to reduce the swelling', which is the worst advice they could be given.

Charcot's osteoarthropathy is usually gradual in onset but can sometimes develop deformity very quickly. A patient who continues to walk on a Charcot foot during the acute onset stage and the stage of bony destruction when the foot is not protected by a cast risks the development of fractures, dislocations, severe deformity, and instability of the affected joints. The Charcot foot can deteriorate with alarming rapidity.

■ Sites affected by Charcot's osteoarthropathy

Charcot's osteoarthropathy usually affects part of the foot or less commonly, the ankle, in people with diabetes. Sites include:

- toes
- forefoot
- midfoot:
  - Lisfranc fracture dislocation
  - medial convexity
  - rocker bottom
- hindfoot: including avulsion of tuberosity of calcaneus
- ankle: unstable ankle mortice
- knee.

It rarely involves the knee: the author has seen five cases in 20 years, and in every case the patient already had bilateral Charcot feet; one patient, in addition, had a Charcot shoulder.

■ Investigations

The following investigations may be needed:

X-ray

- Ankle: straight and lateral views.
- Foot: straight and oblique views.

The importance of having several views to compare cannot be overestimated. It is essential to see straight and lateral views of the ankle, and straight and oblique views of the foot. The extra exposure to X-rays that multiple views entail is minimal and insignificant.

If the Charcot foot is caught early the X-ray may be normal. The podiatrist should look for increased joint spaces, particularly around the bases of the first and second metatarsals (Fig. 7.3A) The podiatrist should look carefully around the outline of each individual foot bone in turn, looking for crumbles, cracks, fragmentation, dislocations and increased joint spaces. Periostial thickening along the shafts of the metatarsals (Fig. 7.3B), and 'sucked candy' appearances (Fig. 7.3C) are common findings in the neuropathic foot and are not associated with the Charcot process. If the X-ray does not confirm the diagnosis, a bone scan should be ordered.

Bone scan

This is a very sensitive test. Technetium biphosphonate solution is injected into an arm vein and taken up by inflamed areas within the bone, where, on scanning, 2 hours later, it is revealed by darker patches indicating the presence of inflamed bone (Fig. 7.4).

MRI scan/CT scan

These may be helpful when distinguishing between infection and Charcot's osteoarthropathy.

Skin temperature

When the patient first presents with a red, hot, swollen foot, the surface temperature on various sites is measured on both feet and compared.

Blood tests

The following blood tests are ordered:

- C-reactive protein (CRP)
- erythrocyte sedimentation rate (ESR)
- full blood count
- serum uric acid (to exclude gout).

Vein scan

If a deep vein thrombosis is suspected, a vein scan is arranged.

Fig. 7.3 (A) Careful scrutiny of this X-ray reveals a little widening of the space between the bases of the first and second metatarsals. A Charcot foot was diagnosed following a bone scan (B) There is periosteal thickening along the shafts of the metatarsals but this is a normal finding in patients with neuropathy. (C) The 'sucked candy' appearance of the 2nd metatarsal is a common finding in patients with neuropathy and previous history of ulceration, and does not indicate a Charcot.

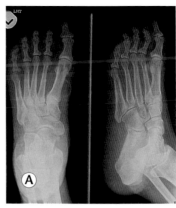

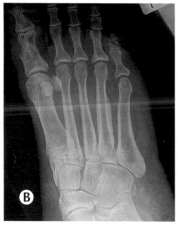

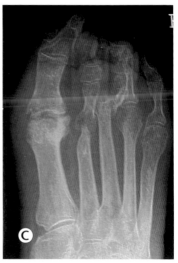

■ Treatment

A total contact cast is applied. The patient receives education on cast care, early detection of danger signs of problems, and the need to attend the clinic immediately problems arise. Patients are given a telephone number to ring in emergency.

Fig. 7.4 The dark areas indicate inflammation. The right foot has acute Charcot's osteoarthropathy. The patient has two fractured toes in the left foot and an area of increased uptake in the midfoot.

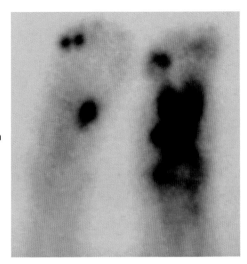

The cast is checked after 1 week. Reduction of oedema may render the cast loose, necessitating application of a fresh cast. The cast is removed in order for the bone scan to be taken, but reapplied at once.

For perfect management, in an ideal world, the affected foot will be completely offloaded in a non-weight-bearing plaster cast for at least 3 months. However, most patients are unable or unwilling to accept this treatment. The problem of persuading patients to accept a cast for a long period is made more difficult because many patients feel no pain in the affected foot and have eyesight that is too poor to see swelling and colour change clearly. Such patients are frequently extremely reluctant to accept a cast, especially when they learn the average length of time they will need treatment will be around 6 months.

The total contact cast (Fig. 7.5) is widely regarded as gold standard treatment of acute Charcot's osteoarthropathy. However, few centres in the UK offer this treatment. This is because:

● Casting is time consuming.
● Casting is labour intensive.
● Casting is regarded as potentially dangerous because problems within the cast may not be detected early.

Fig. 7.5 The patient whose bone scan is shown in Fig. 7.4 is treated with bilateral total contact casts.

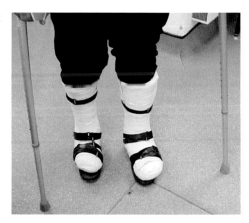

- If patients are non-compliant during the rehabilitation period the foot will relapse.
- A multidisciplinary support team will be necessary for the casting programme.
- Casting is expensive: each cast costs around £40 in materials alone.
- Podiatrists cannot offer total contact casting without support from a physician and an orthotist and the patient's local casualty department, which might need to remove the cast if problems arise out of clinic hours.

Full details of total contact cast manufacture for the treatment of neuropathic ulcers will be found in Chapter 4 on offloading. However, the casting and rehabilitation programme for Charcot patients is different to the programme for patients with ulceration in several ways.

The Charcot patient remains in the cast until the temperature of the two feet are within 1°C and an X-ray shows consolidation of any bony destruction. If the foot and leg have no ulcers or other breaks in the skin, there is no need for antibiotics to be prescribed.

If bony prominences develop, which apply pressures on overlying soft tissues, then ulceration or necrosis will develop which is hard to heal (Fig. 7.6A). Severe infection can destroy the Charcot foot very quickly (Fig. 7.6B).

Fig. 7.6 (A) This patient developed a bony prominence which ulcerated due to pressure from an unsuitable shoe. Ulcers on the Charcot foot are very difficult to heal. (B) When ulcers on the Charcot foot become infected they can destroy the foot with alarming rapidity. This patient's calcaneus collapsed and he came to a major amputation.

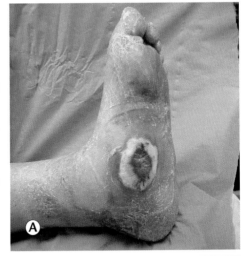

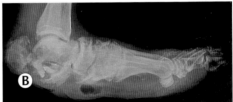

The cast is changed regularly, and each cast should not be left on for longer than 1 month. At cast change, temperature measurements are taken. For these, it is necessary for the patient first to be left with both legs elevated and uncovered for 15 minutes after the cast has been removed: if this is not done the leg that was wrapped in the cast will always be hotter than the other leg.

■ Resolution

Once the temperature of the two feet is within 1°C, at all sites measured, another X-ray is taken for comparison with the initial X-ray.

Once the foot begins to settle down it is essential that the patient continues to rest, and when he enters the rehabilitation phase he

Case study

A 53-year-old man with type 2 diabetes, severe retinopathy, and neuropathy, developed end-stage renal failure and was treated with renal transplantation. He was taking ciclosporin A, azathioprine, and prednisolone to prevent rejection of the kidney. He planned a holiday in the Channel Islands and attended the clinic for a foot check the day before he left; all was well. Two weeks later he returned from holiday with a red, hot, swollen left foot. X-ray revealed acute Charcot's osteoarthropathy with a Lisfranc fracture dislocation. He was not aware of having injured the foot and the only unusual activity he had undertaken was walking on cobbled pavements during his holiday. He had noted a little swelling of the foot by evening, towards the end of the holiday.

Case study

A 72-year-old man with type 2 diabetes and a long history of neuropathic ulceration arrived at the foot clinic for his routine 2-weekly appointment and mentioned that his left foot was a little swollen. Examination revealed a Lisfranc fracture dislocation. The foot was already severely deformed with a medial convexity and bony prominence complicated by necrosis. He had first noticed the problem the previous day.

should only start walking again with considerable caution to avoid re-triggering the Charcot process.

It usually takes at least 6 months for a Charcot foot to settle down, and in patients who are not willing to rest and to follow advice, the destructive process often takes much longer than 6 months to resolve and many patients are left with severe deformity (Fig. 7.7). In some patients the Charcot foot will remain hotter than the non-Charcot foot.

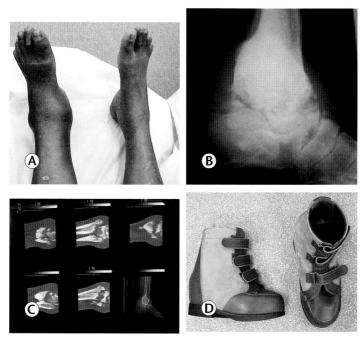

Fig. 7.7 (A) Severe deformity of the left ankle in a lady from Africa whose Charcot joint had not previously been treated. (B) X-ray of the Charcot ankle shown in (A). (C) MRI scan of the Charcot ankle shown in (A). (D) Bespoke boots provided to support the ankle.

■ Residual deformity

The two most common types of major deformity are:

● medial convexity deformity
● rocker-bottom deformity.

However, some patients develop deformity of toes or forefoot, or Charcot's osteoarthropathy of the ankle, which needs particularly careful management to avoid the development of 'flail ankle'.

Studies have been performed to find out whether intravenous infusion of pamidronate (a bisphosphonate and an inhibitor of osteoclast activity) might reduce bony destruction. Trials with oral bisphosphonates are underway.

Patients with severe pain can be given non-steroidal anti-inflammatory agents.

A patient who has had one Charcot foot is at very high risk of developing another. All patients with a history of Charcot should have their feet regularly checked for danger signs of redness, warmth and swelling.

Rehabilitation

If bony consolidation is satisfactory, the orthotist sees the patient, together with the rest of the team, and short-term and long-term management plans are agreed with the patient. These may involve:

- shoes
- insoles
- AFO
- CROW
- Aircast or other brace.

Once the appropriate footwear has been ordered the patient remains in a total contact cast until it is ready, has been fitted, and is deemed acceptable by the team. The patient is rehabilitated as follows:

- The cast is converted into a bivalved removable cast (Fig. 7.8A)
- The patient takes five steps in the new footwear on the first day.
- At the end of the day, and the next morning, the patient's foot is checked for redness, warmth, or swelling.
- If all is well, the patient can take ten steps.
- If all is well, the patient can increase walking by five steps a day, in the house, until the end of the first week.
- If all is well, the patient can continue with gradually increased periods of walking both inside the house and outside.

Chapter 4 describes in detail the different offloading techniques that may be appropriate for the Charcot patient, including bespoke shoes, boots, and externally applied methods of stabilizing the foot and ankle, including the CROW (Fig. 7.8B), AFO (Fig. 7.9) and Aircast (Fig. 7.10).

Surgery

Sometimes, external stabilization is insufficient, particularly in cases of flail ankle, and heroic surgical procedures to pin and plate the foot

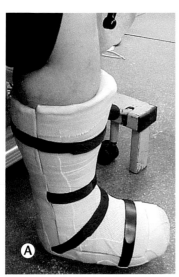 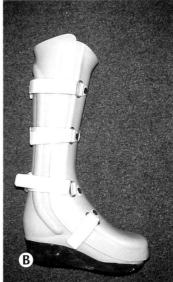

Fig. 7.8 (A) The total contact cast can be bivalved for easy removal during the rehabilitation phase. It is held on with Velcro straps. (B) The Charcot restraint orthotic walker (CROW) is a bivalved bespoke device providing external fixation for unstable Charcot joints.

or ankle may be undertaken (Fig. 7.11). Charcot's osteoarthropathy is very difficult to treat surgically and sometimes the only way to salvage the unstable foot is by internal fixation. A common problem is that screws do not fix well into crumbling weakened bone and frequently work loose.

Patients who undergo this kind of surgery usually need to be kept non-weight bearing for at least 6 months postoperatively, and few orthopaedic surgeons in the United Kingdom are prepared to undertake it.

Some foot surgeons are now using Iliarizov frames to stabilize Charcot ankles, enabling the patient to mobilize much earlier.

Indolent ulcers complicating Charcot's osteoarthropathy may sometimes be treated surgically by exostectomy (removal of the bony prominence underlying an ulcer).

Fig. 7.9 The ankle foot orthosis (AFO).

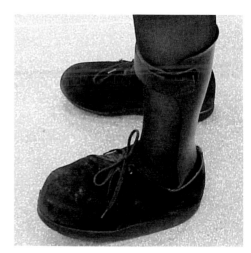

Painful Charcot foot

Thirty per cent of patients complain of pain at the time that they develop acute Charcot's osteoarthropathy, and some complain later of chronic pain after the acute phase has settled, which may trouble them for many years.

PAINFUL NEUROPATHY

Acute painful neuropathy is a singularly disagreeable complication of diabetes. Patients develop severe burning pain and contact discomfort, which is usually in a stocking distribution affecting both feet and legs. They might also complain of sudden stabbing pains (lightning pains), muscular aching, tingling, restlessness, and inability to sleep at night. The pain or discomfort is usually worse at night, and may prevent patients from getting off to sleep, or wake them frequently. Sometimes the pain is so acute that patients are unable to wear normal clothes or to bear the weight of bedclothes at night.

Many patients with acute painful neuropathy have poorly controlled diabetes; however, a particular form of painful neuropathy – insulin neuritis – can develop shortly after glycaemic control has been greatly improved.

Fig. 7.10 The Aircast.

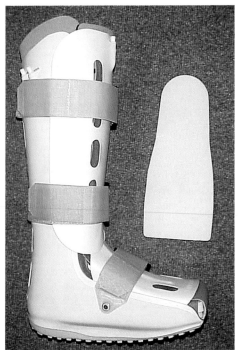

In patients with acute painful neuropathy there are usually no external signs that anything is wrong, but some patients report weight loss which commenced before the pain began. Sometimes the combination of pain and weight loss is regarded as ominous and patients undergo extensive investigations to exclude a malignancy.

Many patients receive little sympathy or support from healthcare professionals because there are no signs that anything is wrong: only a complaining patient. The only good news about painful neuropathy is that it very nearly always gets better within 2 years. Sometimes the pain is superseded by numbness.

■ Aims of treatment

The aim of treatment is to tide patients over for a period of several months, until the pain begins to improve. Reassurance that they will

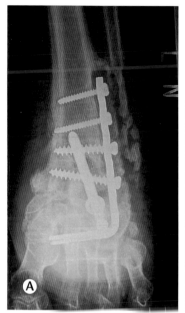
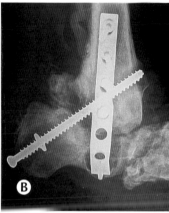

Fig. 7.11 (A) Internal fixation – this unstable Charcot joint has been pinned and plated by an orthopaedic surgeon. (B) Internal fixation – the screw shown in this X-ray later worked loose, tented the overlying skin, and needed surgical removal. However, bony consolidation had occurred: the patient did well, and is walking with an AFO 7 years on.

recover is essential. Patients should be told that many different treatments can be tried. Simple practical physical treatment options include use of a bed cradle to prevent the bedclothes from pressing on the legs at night and keeping a bowl of cool water to splash on the feet if the patient wakes in pain. One of the author's patients found that wearing silk pajamas under day clothes to prevent coarse fabrics from irritating the skin was very helpful. OpSite film or spray may be applied to sensitive areas. A TENS machine can be tried (Fig. 7.12).

Good glycaemic control is essential and all patients with suboptimal control should have an urgent appointment with the diabetes specialist nurse or physician. Topical capsaicin cream helps

Fig. 7.12   This TENS machine may help patients with acute painful neuropathy.

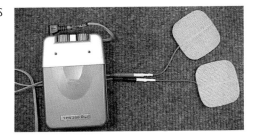

some patients. This product is derived from hot chili peppers and releases substance P: it can take several weeks to improve pain and transitory stinging may occur. After applying capsaicin, patients should wash their hands before touching any sensitive parts of the body.

■ Systemic drugs

Systemic drugs used to treat painful neuropathy include:

- simple analgesics
- hypnotics to help the patient to sleep
- tricyclic antidepressants
- anticonvulsants (gabapentin is frequently prescribed)
- antiarrhythmics.

Evening primrose oil has not been proved to be effective in large clinical trials. There are anecdotal reports that cannabis may be helpful.

In very severe cases, spinal cord stimulation and infusion of intravenous lidocaine may be helpful.

Alternative medicines may have a placebo effect. Acupuncture has been found useful by some patients.

When there has been previous weight loss, the very first sign that the painful neuropathy is resolving can be that the patient starts to regain weight.

At its worst, patients with acute painful neuropathy face an agonizing few months, and it is important for podiatrists to support patients and reassure them that acute painful neuropathy will get better. Patients should be treated kindly and seen frequently.

PATHOLOGICAL FRACTURES

Pathological fractures are very common in the diabetic foot, and the patient is often unaware of the injury because of concurrent neuropathy. Early in the days of the King's foot clinic, one of our research fellows, who was interested in arterial calcification, took X-rays of the hands and feet of a group of patients with neuropathy and ulceration. These were examined retrospectively several years later by another research fellow with an interest in bone density in diabetes, who found that unsuspected fractures were present in 14% of the X-rays. All patients with neuropathy who injure their feet or develop bruising or swelling (Fig 7.13A,B) or pain for no obvious reason (Fig. 7.13C) should undergo X-ray.

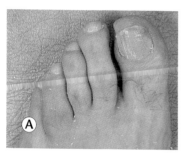

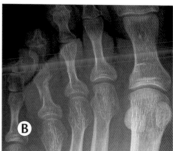

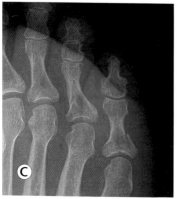

Fig. 7.13 (A) This patient's fourth toe had been swollen for 1 month but she did not seek treatment because the foot was not painful. (B) X-ray of the toe reveals a fracture of the proximal phalanx. (C) This patient's only complaint was of pain: there was no warmth, swelling or bruising but X-ray revealed a fracture of the proximal phalanx of the fifth toe.

Fractures in diabetic feet usually take longer to heal than similar injuries in non-diabetic patients, and the healing time in diabetic neuropaths can be increased two- or three-fold.

Fractures in the diabetic foot should always be taken seriously because they might be the precursors of Charcot's osteoarthropathy. All patients with fractures need careful following and support by an experienced orthopaedic surgeon with an interest in the diabetic foot.

Special care should be taken with casts, providing generous layers of padding at the proximal and distal ends. Exposed toes are liable to be injured when patients have neuropathy and poor vision, so a cast with a closed toe box is useful. Special advice is given to patients never to poke or pour anything down their cast and return rapidly if danger signs arise. The outside of the cast is covered with a layer of stockinette to prevent injury to the other leg from hard sharp fibreglass.

Podiatrists who set up a local programme of casting for managing ulcers, Charcot's osteoarthropathy, or fractures in diabetic neuropathic patients will need local support for the casting programme from diabetes and orthopaedic departments. Patients with neuropathic fractures should be X-rayed again, to confirm that the fracture has stabilized, before casting is discontinued. Rehabilitation after the cast is removed should be gradual; otherwise a Charcot process may be triggered.

Unfortunately, it seems to be common practice in some fracture clinics and casualty departments for young, inexperienced physicians or surgeons to examine a neuropathic foot with painless fracture and to announce that casting is not necessary because the patient can walk without pain.

Neuropathy, renal disease, taking steroids, long duration of diabetes, and type 1 diabetes, all render the diabetic foot patient particularly susceptible to fractures.

8 Wound care

He's a disease that must be cut away.
O he's a limb that has but a disease;
Mortal to cut it off; to cure it easy ...

William Shakespeare, Coriolanus III. II. 293

Wound care has a long and fascinating history. Some of the wound-care products widely used in the past are now regarded as positively detrimental. Hippocrates applied wine to wounds. In the Middle Ages, wounds were cauterized with boiling oil and red-hot irons. In the nineteenth century, Joseph Lister pioneered the use of carbolic acid as an antiseptic. It is interesting to speculate about what future generations will do to wounds, and what they will think of twenty-first century wound care. Will 'moist wound healing' and the science of 'tissue viability' stand up to rigorous scrutiny down the ages, and will podiatrists of the future deplore or deride some of the things podiatrists do to diabetic feet in the early twenty-first century?

WOUND CARE TERMINOLOGY

There are areas of imprecision and overlap in the world of wound care when it comes to describing non-viable tissue. The following definitions are applied within this book:

- *Callus/hyperkeratosis*: an excessively thickened, closely adherent, area of stratum corneum, which has accumulated over an area of the foot subjected to excessive mechanical forces.
- *Granulation tissue*: present in a healing wound and forms a layer of pink or red rosettes.
- *Fibrin*: forms a soft, rubbery, pink- or brownish-apricot-coloured layer over the surface of some wounds. It is semi-translucent and often covers a bed of granulation tissue.
- *Crust*: consists of a piece of dried serum or exudate covering or surrounding a wound.

- *Scab*: a collection of dried blood and fibrin, which forms on the surface of most injuries, covers a healing wound, and is usually red, brown or black and hard in consistency.
- *Slough*: soft, non-viable tissue in a wound. Its components are an amalgam of dead tissue, exudate, previously shed cells and bacteria, which forms on the surface of currently or previously infected or ischaemic wounds. Slough varies in colour and consistency. It may be white, cream, yellow, green, dull red, purple, brown or black. It is soft and may be liquescent and very mobile and loose, hanging by a thread, so to speak, or firm in consistency and adhering to the base of the wound. Slough is associated with unhealing wounds.
- *Eschar*: forms when slough or necrosis on the surface of a wound has dried out and become hard, dark brown or black, with a leathery appearance and consistency.
- *Sequaestrum*: is a piece of dead bone within a wound which in the beginning is firmly attached to healthy bone but gradually loosens and can eventually be lifted out of the wound.
- *Necrosis and gangrene*: are dead tissue, and are dark brown or black in colour. The terms are broadly interchangeable but gangrene is usually regarded as 'worse' than necrosis. Some practitioners refer to gangrene only when the dead tissue is full-thickness and extensive, and refer to more superficial gangrene as necrosis. Many patients find the term 'gangrene' very frightening.
- *Demarcation line*: the border between dry gangrene and normal tissue.

Several different types of tissue can be present in one wound, as can be seen in Fig. 8.1, which shows a wound on the foot of a diabetic patient in end-stage renal failure.

FASHIONS IN WOUND CARE

There are definite 'fashions' in wound care and it is important for podiatrists not to get carried away by the latest flavour-of-the-month-dressing or by the extravagant claims of pharmaceutical representatives and wound product manufacturers. At the time of writing, 'wound bed preparation', vacuum-assisted wound closure (Vac Pump) and antimicrobial dressings containing silver are in vogue; next year it will probably be something new. Fish skin, extract of frog mucus,

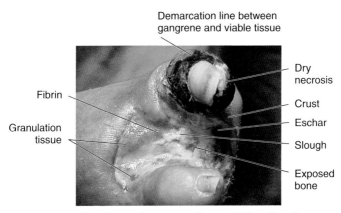

Demarcation line between
gangrene and viable tissue

Dry
necrosis

Fibrin

Crust

Granulation
tissue

Eschar

Slough

Exposed
bone

Fig. 8.1 Wound beds are often not uniform: this foot has dry necrosis, eschar, slough, fibrin, exposed bone and granulation tissue, and a good demarcation line between gangrene and viable tissue.

sugar, honey, Marmite, and topical insulin have all been used on wounds, despite lack of evidence as to their efficacy. Podiatrists should not get carried away by glossy brochures and overenthusiastic reports that are not based on good science and properly conducted studies.

There are problems, too, with some of the terminology used to describe wounds and treatments, much lifted from the world of nursing and tissue viability, which appears to have little basis in science. One thing is certain: there is no panacea for the diabetic foot when it comes to wound care.

Treatments for wounds include:

- debridement
- dressings
- advanced wound products (high-tech interventions).

However, in addition to using woundcare techniques, it is essential for podiatrists not to overlook the importance of also establishing mechanical, metabolic, vascular, educational, and microbiological control (all of which are fully covered elsewhere in this book).

Good wound care alone will not heal the majority of indolent diabetic foot ulcers. Some modern dressings are extremely expensive, and so is the time of the staff who do the dressings, and many advanced treatments are prohibitively costly. Many 'problem' wounds may be hard to heal only because very basic aspects of wound management have not been dealt with.

THE TIMESCALE TO HEALING: WHAT IS 'DELAYED WOUND HEALING'?

Uncomplicated neuropathic ulcers, given good multidisciplinary care by an experienced team, should be healing well within 6 weeks. If they are not, then something has gone wrong with previous or current care.

Around 70% of uncomplicated ischaemic ulcers caught early and given optimal conservative care by a multidisciplinary team should be improving or healed within 15 weeks. If they are not starting to heal well within this time period then something has gone wrong with previous or current care.

There is a need for very regular review of the state of the wound and the healing rate.

CLOSING THE 'WINDOW OF OPPORTUNITY'

If ulcers are taking longer than usual to heal, then it is usually because some aspect of their care is not being fully addressed. There may be rare and complex reasons for the non-healing of wounds but, all too often, some very basic aspects of taking control have been neglected.

'Cut and come again' is the bane of the podiatry profession. When working with high-risk patients, podiatrists cannot afford to sit back and wait while their patients fail to heal and their ulcers enter a state of chronicity. Podiatrists must take active steps to improve care and speed healing. This often means turning to other healthcare professionals for advice or support, and podiatrists should always seek help from other members of the multidisciplinary diabetic foot team early rather than late. Podiatrists should not work in isolation and must always remember that with every ulcer there is a 'window of opportunity' to achieve early healing. This window will close if early treatment is suboptimal and healthcare professionals are complaisant about healing failure.

SHARED CARE

A situation sometimes arises when community podiatrists hold on to patients with ulcers because they enjoy treating ulcers and do not wish to refer the patient on and 'lose' him to the hospital team (Fig. 8.2). This can have disastrous outcomes for the high-risk diabetic foot patient. The ideal situation is a shared care programme where the patient is managed jointly by community and hospital, the community podiatrist is not 'de-skilled', and the patient is not lost by either party, but benefits from shared care. Another way of overcoming the problem is by organizing regular training rotations where community podiatrists are able to spend some time working in the hospital with the multidisciplinary diabetic foot team.

The dangers of impaired and delayed wound healing include:

- osteomyelitis
- rapidly spreading soft tissue infection

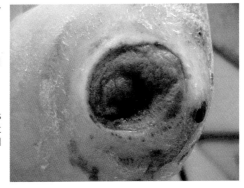

Fig. 8.2 A community podiatrist treated this neuropathic ulcer with debridement of callus, felt padding and dressings for nearly 6 months. It was not until the wound had developed a deep sinus and osteomyelitis that the patient was referred to the hospital diabetic foot clinic. The window of opportunity for achieving rapid healing had been lost and the foot took 9 months to heal. The NICE guidelines say that ulcers should be rapidly referred to multidisciplinary diabetic foot clinics.

- gangrene
- amputation
- destruction of fibrofatty padding and formation of scar tissue, which renders the patient susceptible to further ulceration
- possible long-term health hazards related to raised inflammatory products and high fibrinogen levels associated with injury and infection.

ADJUNCTIVE CARE FOR PATIENTS WITH DIABETIC FOOT WOUNDS

As already said, good wound care alone will not heal ulcers. Adjunctive care is also needed (Box 8.1).

Box 8.1   Adjunctive care

Education in wound care

Patients need to be made aware that foot ulcers are a very serious health problem, even if they are not painful. They should be told that a few days of total rest and offloading in the early stages of an ulcer can often arrest its development and prevent weeks, months, years, or a lifetime of disability. Almost every indolent ulcer begins with a small problem that is neglected or given inappropriate care, and delayed or inadequate treatment can lead to disaster.

Patients whose ulcers heal should be warned that they are at high-risk of future problems and offered regular treatment if necessary. They should be reminded to check their feet every day for the danger signs of actual or impending foot problems because relapse is very common. Patients with ulcers should be taught wound care and the signs that an ulcer is deteriorating. They should be encouraged to rest, to take time off work, if possible, and not to go on holiday until their foot problem has resolved (see Chapter 9).

Offloading

Dr RD Lawrence, who founded the first diabetic clinic in the United Kingdom at King's College Hospital and was himself diabetic, insisted that any of his patients with a foot problem should rest in bed and use crutches to totally offload the affected foot. This is ideal advice: however, in the real world this approach may be impractical and cannot be used long-term; Chapter 4 on offloading offers alternative approaches.

Vascular control

Patients with pulseless feet and ischaemic ulcers need formal vascular assessment and possible vascular intervention if the ABPI is below 0.5 (see Chapter 6). If the patient is critically ischaemic there is no time to waste on a trial of whether healing will occur because gangrene can develop very rapidly.

Metabolic control

Optimal control of hyperglycaemia, hypertension, hyperlipidaemia and smoking is essential for all diabetic patients (see Chapter 2). It is likely that hyperglycaemic patients will be particularly susceptible to infection. Cardiac and kidney problems need to be treated. Oedema can delay wound healing.

Microbiological control

Infection is a great destroyer of diabetic feet. Early detection and aggressive treatment of infection are essential (see Chapter 5).

DEBRIDEMENT

Podiatric debridement is sharp debridement which involves:

- Removal of callus from pressure points on the sole of the neuro-pathic foot (Fig. 8.3) and, more rarely from the margins of the neuroischaemic foot (Fig. 8.4), or from other sites of previous ulceration on both types of foot.
- Sharp debridement of callus, slough, undermined edges and non-viable material from around, upon and within neuropathic ulcers (see Fig. 8.3) and from around ischaemic ulcers (see Fig. 8.4).
- Sharp debridement of gangrene.

Other methods of achieving debridement are:

- debridement with maggots (larva therapy)
- physical debridement
- enzymatic debridement

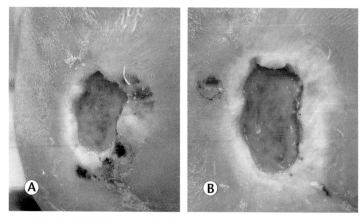

Fig. 8.3 (A) Debridement of callus is essential to achieve healing of this neuropathic ulcer. (B) Callus has been debrided from around the ulcer. At 10 o'clock a small haemorrhage has been caused. This will not be a problem as the neuropathic foot has a good blood supply.

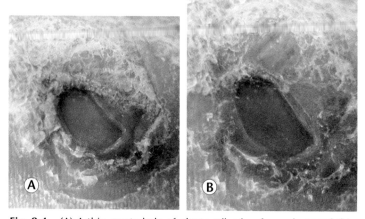

Fig. 8.4 (A) A thin crusty halo of glassy callus has formed around this marginated ischaemic ulcer. The wound bed is pale and the surrounding skin looks ischaemic. A vascular assessment should be undertaken immediately. (B) The ischaemic ulcer has been debrided. Great care has been taken not to damage surrounding skin. Hard crusty accretions of tissue, which might catch on dressings and cause trauma, have been cut away.

- chemical debridement, including acid and caustic preparations, some 'folk remedies', and over-the-counter proprietary products
- debridement with dressings.

However, many of these techniques are not at all suitable for the diabetic foot.

■ Sharp debridement

Sharp debridement is probably the most important treatment that podiatrists can offer their diabetic foot patients. Sharp debridement is by far the quickest, most efficient, most effective and safest – in careful and expert hands – method of debridement. Although other techniques will also be briefly discussed later in the chapter, this is often only to emphasize their unsuitability for the diabetic foot.

Regular sharp debridement is essential treatment for the ulcerated, infected, or necrotic diabetic foot. It is a key aspect of wound care for the diabetic foot, speeding healing, preventing deterioration, and enabling accurate clinical and microbiological assessment to take place.

It is important to understand why sharp debridement is such a necessary and effective treatment so that the procedure can be explained and justified to patients and other healthcare professionals, who are often critical because they do not understand the role of the podiatrist.

Advantages of sharp debridement

- Enables quick removal of non-viable material (the presence of which promotes infection because it is an ideal growth medium for bacteria).
- Gives access to previously inaccessible areas.
- Reveals the true depths of a lesion (Fig. 8.5).
- Reduces pressure from neglected callus.
- Enables wounds to drain freely.
- Enables the taking of deep tissue samples or swabs for microscopy and culture. Organisms grown from material taken from the depths of the ulcer are less likely to be superficial contaminants.
- Does not change the colour and texture of the wound bed, therefore rendering assessment easier.
- Changes an indolent ulcer into an acute ulcer.

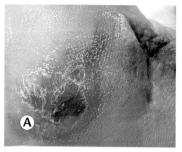

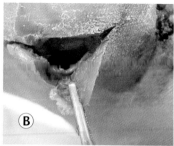

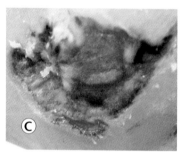

Fig. 8.5 (A) Until debridement has been performed it is impossible to assess this neuropathic foot with a thick, discoloured callus. (B) Initial stages of debridement reveal a cavity beneath the callus. (C) Callus has been debrided away to reveal a neuropathic ulcer.

Disadvantages of sharp debridement

● Can cause inadvertent damage to the ischaemic foot.
● Sensitive ischaemic ulcers can be painful when debrided.
● May cause excessive bleeding.
● Inexperienced practitioners might go too far and cause damage.
● Knowledge of anatomy is needed.
● Danger of accidentally cutting operator or patient.
● Need for careful disposal of scalpel blades.
● Need for instrument sterilization service.

Instruments for sharp debridement

The instruments used for sharp debridement include:

● scalpel handle and blades
● forceps
● probe (one arm of the forceps can be used instead)
● scissors

- tissue nippers
- specialized instruments such as bone cutters for experienced clinicians who have been trained in their use.

The use of disposable 'throw-away' instruments for debriding is not recommended. Plastic-handled disposable scalpels are poorly balanced and become blunt quickly: plastic forceps are clumsy and imprecise and do not grip well. Good quality instruments stand up well to frequent sterilization, are easier to use, and minimize the possibility of repetitive stress injuries in the operator.

Dressings packs containing sterile gauze, and Galipot and sterile field are useful. The tools needed for sharp debridement should be available in a basic ulcer pack, which is preferably centrally sterilized, and contains scalpel handle, Adson Brown untoothed forceps and blunt sharp scissors. Supplies of non-shedding gauze, saline, dressings, tape and bandages are also needed. The scalpel handle holds a disposable scalpel blade. Most practitioners use an E11, a D10 or a D15 blade for debriding.

The need for postgraduate experience in sharp debridement of high-risk feet

Unfortunately, many podiatry schools in the United Kingdom do not teach sharp debridement of the diabetic foot adequately (apart from simple callus removal), because they lack access to sufficient high-risk patients with foot ulcers. Clinicians may therefore need to gain postgraduate experience in practical ulcer management. Although there are many illustrations of feet before and after debridement in this book, the reader will find that just as one picture is worth a thousand words, seeing a real-life debridement is far more useful than merely seeing a series of 'before, during and after' pictures. Further practical experience can be gained by:

- visiting large, hospital-based diabetic foot clinics
- sitting in with clinical specialists, more advanced practitioners, surgeons and surgical podiatrists
- visiting specialist woundcare centres
- going into the operating theatre with surgeons.

Many multidisciplinary diabetic foot clinics now offer training rotations to community podiatrists and welcome visitors from all healthcare professions.

Knowledge of anatomy is necessary

Podiatrists planning to sharp-debride high-risk diabetic feet may need to update their knowledge of anatomy. Useful texts include photographs of dissections, such as the 2nd edition of McMinn, Hutchings and Logan's *Colour Atlas of Foot and Ankle Anatomy* (published by Mosby in 1996).

Sharp debridement of callus

The only safe way to remove callus from a diabetic foot is by sharp debridement with scalpel and forceps. Most practitioners use an E11 scalpel blade or a D10 blade: they are equally effective.

A plaque of callus should not be removed in one piece but rather in thin slickets, while the area being operated on is stretched by the fingers of the operator's free hand. This applies tension to the skin, immobilizes the area being treated, and enables even removal of the callus. If skin tension is not applied the area being cut moves with the motions of the scalpel, rendering operating more difficult.

The podiatrist can tell how deep it is safe to go in removal of callus by a combination of visual and tactile clues. There is a difference in the texture of callus and the underlying tissue. The callus is firmer and the blade slides through it more easily. The deeper the callus is situated, the more moisture it holds. If a plaque of callus is very thick, the deeper areas of the plaque become macerated. This macerated callus is very deceptive as the difference in texture between macerated callus and underlying tissue is decreased. It may be helpful to stop working on a macerated area and move to another area needing treatment and return to the original area after a few minutes, when the surface area will have dried out and the difference in texture between the surface and the underlying area will be more apparent and the operator will be less likely to go too far and risk removing too much callus and cutting the patient. Fortunately, macerated callus is a whitish colour when compared to non-macerated callus, so there are visual clues also.

The texture and appearance of the area of previously callused skin, after removal of the callus, should be almost indistinguishable from the surrounding area (Fig. 8.6). However, if the callus was very thick it will not be possible to achieve this appearance until the debrided area has dried out.

All podiatrists are familiar with debriding simple callus, and aware that the colour and consistency of callus changes, softening and

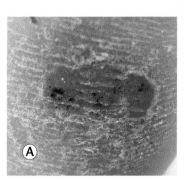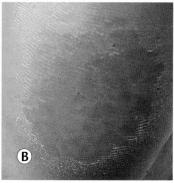

Fig. 8.6 (A) The tiny speckles of blood within this dry plaque of callus on a neuropathic foot are warning signs that the callus is becoming too thick and will lead to ulceration unless it is removed. (B) The plaque of callus has been debrided away, thus preventing a neuropathic ulcer.

becoming whiter and more opaque with increasing depth, particularly when the callus has been allowed to accumulate for a considerable period of time. The colour and consistency of callus will change depending on its fluid content. Callus that is macerated by water, exudate or bodily fluids becomes rubbery in consistency and the surface might take on a corrugated appearance, which recedes as the tissue dries out. Increased water content causes callus to become white and opaque. Callus might also take up colour from shoe dye, blood, or exudate: for example, discharge from an ulcer infected with *Pseudomonas aeruginosa* can cause characteristic blue–green staining of surrounding callus and skin. Generally speaking, the deeper the callus, the higher the water content will be.

External pressure, underlying tissue breakdown and the presence of fluid filled cavities also change the appearance and consistency of callus. A plaque of callus may be divided into several distinct layers where clear serous fluid has seeped into the tissues from an underlying tissue breakdown. Many discrete cavities in callus are found in sites overlying an ulcer cavity, or an area of infection where pus has tracked along planes between layers of tissue. The surface appearances are often very deceptive and it is impossible to determine the true extent of the lesion or the severity of the problem until a full debridement has been performed, all tracts explored and laid open, and the area palpated to ensure that there are no painful areas or pus seeping from a deeper region of the foot.

Contents of recesses and cavities in callus and epidermis range from clear fluid, serosanguinous fluid, jelly-like fibrin, frank pus, and white, cream, yellow or pinkish material of a pasty consistency, which may be made up of epidermal cell debris. An amber coloured area in callus (Fig. 8.7A) is often a sign of underlying ulceration (Fig. 8.7B) with accumulation of serous or serosanguinous fluid.

Great care should always be taken when removing callus from ischaemic feet. Although heavy callus formation is unusual in diabetic neuroischaemic feet, plaques of thin, glassy callus sometimes develop on the plantar surface of the forefoot, on the medial and lateral borders of the foot, and on and around the heel. Ischaemic callus is very slippery and hard and great care must be taken not to cut the patient by mistake, and not to remove too much callus. It should always be remembered that any injury to the neuroischaemic foot can lead to ulceration. Spraying the foot with spirit to dampen callus enables subtle variations in depth and structure, skin striations and other small features to be seen more clearly.

In the United Kingdom, all podiatrists are taught to remove callus from skin that is stretched by the fingers of one hand while callus is removed with a scalpel held by the other hand. This technique maintains 'skin tension', thus enabling smooth and even removal of callus.

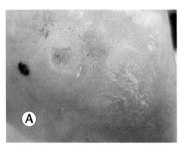 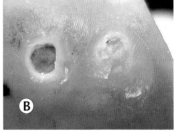

Fig. 8.7 (A) Appearances can be deceptive. The only indication of an underlying ulcer is an area of callus which is a darker colour than other plaques of callus. (B) The callus has been debrided away to reveal a neuropathic ulcer.

However, many podiatrists have never been taught the simple technique of using a pair of forceps, instead of the fingers of the other hand, to maintain tension in the material being operated on.

Scalpel and forceps technique

When debriding slough from wounds, wet necrosis, and macerated callus, the author has found the 'scalpel and forceps' debridement technique (which uses forceps for applying tension to tissues that are cut away with a sterile scalpel) is the most quick and precise way of removing non-viable tissue.

A pair of Adson Brown non-toothed forceps is the recommended type of forceps. When working with slippery material it is easier to get a grip with untoothed forceps. The slender arm of the forceps can be used as a probe (Fig. 8.8A) to assess the depth and degree of undermining of the ulcer (undermining being the area where an ulcer burrows under apparently intact surrounding skin at the edge of the ulcer) and to explore any sinuses in the base of the wound.

The forceps are used to pick up, and apply gentle traction to, the material being cut away (Fig. 8.8B). This maintains tension and

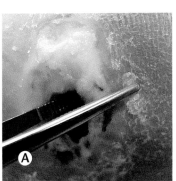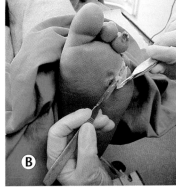

Fig. 8.8 (A) Adson Brown untoothed forceps are a useful tool. Here they are used as a probe, which is passed under surrounding skin to demonstrate 'undermining' where the ulcer has burrowed under the skin. (B) The forceps grasp the tissue to be cut away, applying gentle traction, which enables the operator to dissect with more precision and less likelihood of cutting the patient.

makes it far easier to dissect with precision, and blades keep sharper for longer than if they are cutting slack tissue. The untoothed forceps give far more flexibility and a far better grip than toothed forceps. Locking artery forceps are not recommended because the piece of material being picked up will change frequently, and constantly locking and unlocking artery forceps is tiring.

Management of crusts and scabs
Dry crusts and scabs can often be left in place unless they are projecting from the surface, when a scalpel can pare them down to prevent trauma if they get caught on dressings or socks. They should be kept covered with a dry dressing until fully healed.

Sharp debridement of slough
Be it called slough, eschar, necrosis or gangrene, non-viable tissue is best removed from wounds by attaching the forceps, applying gentle traction and gently dissecting away until as much as possible of the non-viable material has been removed (Fig. 8.9). If slough is extremely wet, slimy, and slippery it can first be rubbed and dried with sterile dry gauze. This will remove a considerable amount of moisture from the slough, which is then easier to grip with the forceps.

Sharp debridement of eschar
Plaques of dry, leathery eschar on heels with no signs of infection around or beneath them, which are firmly anchored and not mobile,

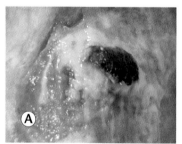
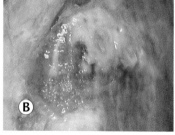

Fig. 8.9   (A) The dark brown eschar, sitting on a cushion of slough, needs to be removed to speed healing of this ulcer. (B) The eschar has been carefully dissected away.

should not be debrided away below the level of the surrounding skin surface. However, if an eschar is sitting on a cushion of moist slough, or is associated with surrounding cellulitis or purulent discharge from the edge, it should be fully debrided.

Dry eschar on heels should not be removed piecemeal, but as a gradual process over several weeks.

Sharp debridement of necrosis and gangrene

This involves removal of dead tissue:

- in the base of an ulcer (may be moist or dry)
- extending from ulcer to involve surrounding tissues (may be moist or dry)
- superficial (may be moist or dry)
- deep (may be moist or dry)
- with clear demarcation line at junction with viable tissue, dry
- with unclear demarcation line at junction with viable tissue, moist.

All moist necrosis in the neuropathic foot needs urgent debridement. This can sometimes be performed as an outpatient procedure but the patient usually needs hospital admission, intravenous antibiotics and surgical debridement. A preliminary debridement in the diabetic foot clinic can yield valuable material for microscopy and culture, as sometimes there is a delay before the patient goes to theatre. As much wet necrotic material as possible should be removed.

DEALING WITH SINUSES AND USE OF A PROBE

Some wound beds are not of a broadly uniform depth, and contain one or more sinuses extending to deeper areas of the foot. Sometimes the sinus is open and sometimes it is sealed off but reveals its presence because the area of wound bed overlying it is a different colour to the rest of the ulcer bed, being usually less pink, or of a greyish or purple hue.

Signs of a sinus include excessive moisture and discharge associated with a convex 'pouting' wound bed with a pucker or crease or slit in the wound bed into which a probe can be inserted. Many ulcers complicated by a sinus have a consistently wet and 'soupy' appearance.

Some clinicians are concerned lest, when inserting a probe in the search for a sinus, they apply excessive force and injure the patient. When probing it is necessary to be gentle, yet firm. In medieval times, a parsley stalk was used as a probe; it buckled if excessive force was applied and thus did not apply sufficient pressure to cause injury.

Practitioners who are nervous or inexperienced at probing wounds should not apply a force of more than 10 g to the probe (and can practice applying a monofilament to the skin until it buckles at a force of 10 g so that they can get a feel for how much pressure they are applying).

■ Rationale for probing wounds

Wounds are probed:

- To help to ascertain the true dimensions of a wound. Many wounds of the diabetic foot look superficial but have hidden depths, often due to uncontrolled pressure or infection.
- To diagnose osteomyelitis. If a probe touches bone, the likelihood is that the patient has osteomyelitis and will need surgery or long-term antibiotics (see Chapter 5).

MANAGEMENT OF ULCERS

■ Warning signs

Warning signs and symptoms that an ulcer is imminent include:

- red or blue marks
- blisters
- discoloration around a fissure
- speckles of bleeding within callus is a warning sign that pressure is damaging the underlying tissues
- blistering within callus
- discolouration beneath callus
- hot areas
- cold areas
- painful areas
- moist areas
- following chemical applications (corn cures, etc.).

All these warning signs should be acted on: it is sometimes possible to prevent the lesion from progressing any further with timely intervention.

■ Cause of ulcers

It is essential to investigate the cause of ulcers, and also to distinguish between neuropathic feet and neuroischaemic feet because the management is different.

■ Debridement of neuropathic ulcers

Before starting debridement it is important to ensure that the patient is aware of the need to remove non-viable tissue to speed ulcer healing, and that it may be necessary to cause bleeding if an adequate debridement is to be performed.

The aim is to remove all surrounding callus, slough, necrosis, heaped-up debris, and undermined edges. The material to be removed can be grasped with untoothed Adson Brown forceps and gentle traction applied so that the material being cut away is under tension and thus easier to cut. A small area of callus can be partially cut through and then used as an anchor for the forceps to hold on to.

When callus at the edge of the ulcer is being grasped it should be pulled in the direction of the centre of the ulcer, and lifted upwards and away from the wound bed so that it can be dissected away with less risk of cutting the wound bed.

When debriding the wound bed of a neuropathic ulcer, all healthy granulation tissue (shiny red or pink material with rosettes) should be left alone but as much non-viable material as possible should be removed. However, podiatrists have to decide whether an adequate debridement can be performed in an outpatient setting or whether a surgical debridement would be more suitable.

Some ulcers or wounds have a rubbery translucent layer of pale fawn or light brown fibrin covering them. This can be removed (it pulls off quite easily) or left as desired.

The edges of the wound should be saucerized, which means that there should be a gentle slope from the edge of the surrounding skin down to the wound bed, as there is from the top edge of a saucer to the base where the cup sits. No undermined areas should be left: it should not be possible to pass a probe from the bed of the ulcer underneath the surrounding skin. However, the podiatrist should judge whether undermined areas that need to be removed are so large that this is best done by a surgeon in theatre.

The podiatrist should not worry too much about causing bleeding in the neuropathic foot (within reason!) because this is often unavoidable. However, patients should be forewarned and new patients may need reassurance.

◼ Viable and non-viable tissue

It is important to distinguish between viable and non-viable soft tissue when debriding and the following questions may be asked:

- Is the area pink or red?
- Does it bleed?
- Is it painful when touched?
- Is it firm and smooth?

If the answer is yes, then it is almost certainly viable and should not be debrided away.

◼ Debridement of ischaemic ulcers

Ischaemic ulcers are very different to neuropathic ulcers in their appearance. It is unusual to find exuberant callus formation on an ischaemic foot. Callus, when present, tends to be hard and thin and glassy, and it is rare to see an ulcer under a callus in the neuro-ischaemic diabetic foot.

The ischaemic ulcer usually begins with a red mark that blisters and breaks down into a shallow lesion with a wet, translucent, pale base. The base is often cream or white with very few faint pale granulations. Many ischaemic ulcers quickly form a base of yellow slough, which is closely adherent. There is sometimes a steep slope at the edges (a punched-out appearance), and the foot is generally hairless, with atrophic skin.

The only debridement that should be performed on the ischaemic foot is:

- Removal of the halo of thin hard callus that sometimes develops around an ischaemic ulcer.
- Removal of slough when this can be performed without damage to underlying or surrounding viable tissue.

- Removal of necrosis when this can be undertaken without damage to adjoining or underlying tissue (Fig. 8.10).
- Paring back of nail associated with a subungual ulcer.

◼ Debridement of necrosis and facilitated autoamputation in the neuroischaemic foot

If the foot is very ischaemic then it is not wise to remove a gangrenous toe surgically. Careful and gradual removal of necrotic tissue by the podiatrist speeds healing and renders infection less likely, but should be performed very carefully. If necrosis is dry and firm, then minimal debridement is needed. The demarcation line should be kept clear of accumulated debris and any areas where discharge is apparent should be gently debrided to achieve drainage of associated pockets of pus and to enable taking of a sample for microbiology. If necrosis is wet then as much tissue as possible should be removed, using scalpel and forceps, and sent for microscopy and culture, and antibiotics should be requested.

Toes with full thickness necrosis awaiting autoamputation should be separated from adjoining toes by placing a dry dressing between them. They will gradually become loose and it is often possible to remove a large portion of the gangrenous toe through the inter-

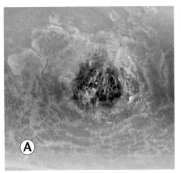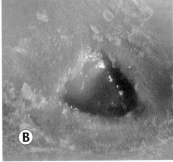

Fig. 8.10   (A) This ischaemic ulcer is covered with a layer of necrosis. Who knows what lies beneath? (B) Careful debridement of necrotic tissue reveals a healthy, granulating wound bed and pearly new epithelium.

phalangeal joint distal to the demarcation line between gangrene and viable tissue (see Chapter 6) leaving a small gangrenous stump that is less likely to be traumatized, and easier to debride and dress, than an excessively mobile entire toe. Patients should always be warned well in advance that when the toe becomes mobile it may be necessary to remove a portion of it to speed healing, and that it may be possible for the podiatrist to remove the entire black toe once it is loose enough.

■ Subungual ulceration

Ulcers frequently develop beneath thickened nails that have been subjected to pressure from the footwear or a trauma. Affected nails may appear excessively thickened, leak moisture from under or around the nail plate, or appear discoloured. Ulceration beneath the nail is often hard to assess until the nail is gently pared back to reveal one of the following:

- a cavity containing serous fluid with a pale pink base
- a cavity containing pus with a red base
- a cavity containing liquid or clotted blood
- a cavity containing dried out exudate or dry blood.

An area of necrosis, which may be wet or dry, or exposed phalanx, might also be present. It is often impossible to distinguish between subungual blood and subungual necrosis unless the nail plate is cut back.

Management of subungual ulcer

The nail plate overlying the defect should be cut back with nippers or gently pared away with a scalpel.

The contents of any cavity should be evacuated and the base of the lesion inspected. After cleaning with saline, cover with a dressing, and treat as appropriate for neuropathic ulcer or ischaemic ulcer.

Sometimes the nail plate is cut back to expose a healed nail bed under dried callus or blood from a previous ulcer or injury.

Care should be taken not to leave rough or proud areas of nail behind, which may catch on dressings or socks.

Ischaemic ulcers often develop a little halo of hard dry callus, which is best removed because it can catch on dressings or footwear and cause trauma to adjoining tissues.

■ Onychocryptosis

The classic ingrowing toenail or onychocryptosis is often the result of incorrect cutting of the nails. Patients with impaired vision or poor dexterity may inadvertently leave behind a section of uncut nail and, as the nail plate grows forward, the uncut spike at the edge of the nail is forced sideways into the nail sulcus. Once the skin is penetrated there is a foreign-body reaction with formation of granulation tissue, and failure to heal until the spike of nail is removed. Proprietary remedies are of little use. Infection is a common complication.

Ingrowing toe nails can also be caused by tight shoes pressing on the side of the toe, or by a 'one-off' trauma, such as from walking barefoot and stubbing the toe, or dropping a heavy object on the foot.

Patients with a very broad, thin nail plate and a fleshy nail sulcus are especially prone to develop onychocryptosis, which presents as:

- a painful nail sulcus: pressure from the nail edge may have caused onychophosis (corn or callus or debris in the sulcus)
- infection down the side of the nail
- granulation tissue
- discharge.

The nail sulcus is explored with a probe, or the blunt side of a D15 blade, until the splinter of nail is located. A small wedge is removed from the side of the nail, incorporating the splinter. The operator works by cutting through the nail plate, working distal to proximal and taking great care not to cause further tissue damage by penetrating the sulcus or the nail bed. When removing the wedge it is important to ascertain the direction in which the spike of nail is growing into the flesh, as careless removal will cause further tissue damage. It is usually necessary to lift the loose piece out, moving it proximally and away from the sulcus, to free the splinter from the flesh of the sulcus, and then, when it is clear that the spike is free, moving the wedge and spike distally until it can be lifted away.

It is useful education to show the wedge and spike to the patient and talk to him about how the problem was caused.

In patients whose neuropathy is not profound, the above procedure may sometimes be uncomfortable but the pain felt is less than would be felt if a local anaesthetic was administered. (Patients are, however, well advised not to watch the procedure, as those who watch war films might find that it reminds them of torture scenes.)

If the problem cannot be controlled by the above intervention the patient should be referred for nail surgery. However, it is essential that, before any invasive procedure is undertaken, a full neurological and vascular assessment is performed, and that regular follow up occurs until full healing has occurred. If the toe is ischaemic, the patient should be seen by the vascular team before any management decisions are made.

It has been our policy at King's to prescribe prophylactic antibiotics to all diabetic feet undergoing nail surgery.

Onychocryptosis can be acute or chronic, when there is associated hypergranulation. Some podiatrists like to treat hypergranulation tissue with silver nitrate to reduce it, but the author has never found this necessary as hypergranulation tissue clears up once the irritating nail spike has been removed and infection is controlled. Topical caustic applications to diabetic feet are always best avoided.

BLISTERS

Causes of blisters include frictional forces, pressure, oedema, thermal injuries, contact with noxious chemicals, and systemic disease.

Many diabetic foot problems, including burns, puncture wounds, neuropathic ulcers, ischaemic ulcers, and infections might first present as a blister. Without inspecting the wound base, it can sometimes be difficult to make a diagnosis. Blisters vary in size and consistency as follows, and may be:

- small (under 1 cm) and flaccid
- small and tense
- large (over 1 cm) and flaccid
- large and tense.

Contents of blisters also vary and include:

- clear fluid
- yellow fluid/serum
- serosanguinous fluid
- liquid blood
- clotted serum
- clotted blood
- purulent discharge

● liquefied tissues broken down by severe infection: this leads to the appearance of purplish blisters or blebs on an infected diabetic foot, which is an ominous sign.

Bases of blisters may be made up of:

● moist intact epithelium
● denuded epithelium
● exposed dermis
● slough
● superficial necrosis (wet or dry)
● partial-thickness necrosis (wet or dry)
● full-thickness necrosis (wet or dry).

The skin surrounding blisters may be:

● normal
● lifting
● discoloured
    ● blue
    ● red
    ● black
● oedematous.

▌ Treatment of blisters

There are two different schools of thought. The first holds that blisters should not be punctured. The rationale for this is that:

● infection can enter the foot through any break in the blister
● the blister forms a natural cushion, which protects the underlying tissues from pressure and friction,
● there will be less pain,
● intact overlying skin is better than any artificial dressing
● healing will be quicker.

The second holds that:

● Unless blisters are very small they are likely to break anyway and rupturing them is best done under sterile conditions.
● If a very large and tense blister is left, then the hydrostatic pressure from the contents under tension may render the base necrotic by preventing blood flow within the capillary bed.
● It is difficult to assess the wound without inspecting its base.

- It may be useful to take a swab of the contents of the bulla for microscopy and culture.

It is not always necessary to deroof an entire blister: a cross can be cut in it (Fig. 8.11) and the quadrants folded back for inspection of the base, which can be cleansed of purulent discharge, examined and probed. (Draining blisters with a hypodermic syringe is not an effective alternative because they refill quickly and the puncture site frequently seals so that drainage stops.)

There are some clear advantages in the second school of thought for diabetic foot patients.

After inspection and decompressing, the blister is cleaned and covered with a sterile dressing and treated as an ulcer until it is fully healed. Sometimes the quarters of skin will readhere to the underlying surface, in which circumstances the blister will heal very quickly. The base of a blister should be cleansed gently because sometimes islets of epithelium are present on the basal dermis and, again, in these circumstances the lesion will heal quicker if the islets are left in place than if they are removed and epithelium has to migrate from the edges to cover the wound.

Old blisters that have dried out present as a hard rough raised area of dry epithelium or callus, which may contain quite a large volume of dried out exudate, serum, or blood. The blister and contents can be gently smoothed off with a scalpel, or removed to reveal an

Fig. 8.11 A cross has been cut in this blister on the apex of a neuropathic toe. This enables the wound bed to be inspected and the wound can drain.

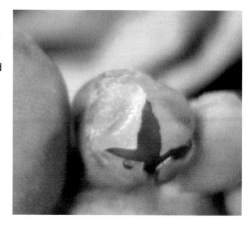

intact base. If rough protruding areas are allowed to remain there is a danger that they will catch on hose and tear underlying tissue: they become rock hard and if subjected to pressure or friction may lead to ulceration. After debridement the area should be covered with a dressing for at least 48 hours, even if it appears to be intact.

Deeper blisters with a necrotic base, which remain free of infection, will dry out to form a leathery plaque or eschar, which can be debrided little by little, over several treatments, to prevent accumulation of debris around the edges. Any areas of eschar that stand proud of the surrounding surface should be gently debrided. As the eschar becomes loose, or if it is sitting upon a cushion of moist slough, it should be gently debrided away. At one time, practitioners would inject a solution of Varidase into an eschar to speed removal: however, this is never recommended for diabetic feet. Nor is the application of topical Varidase or other chemical debriding agents recommended.

If non-viable material is needed for microscopy and culture, it should be taken from the deepest, wettest site, or any area associated with redness, swelling, or purulent discharge. If possible, surface material should be debrided away and only deeper tissues sent for culture to avoid confounding the microbiologist with surface organisms.

FISSURES

Fissures appear in dry skin and in dry callus. Fissures can be superficial or deep, taut or gaping. The podiatrist should carefully examine the edges and sides of the fissures. If they are covered with epithelium this will prevent the fissure from closing and, in the neuropathic foot, if the fissure is deep to the dermis, all callus should be debrided from the sides, and the fissure can then be closed with steristrips. Care should be taken not to seal off the entire length of the fissure with the steristrips, so that drainage of any exudate can occur. Once the fissure has closed and healed, regular applications of emollient will help to render the skin flexible and prevent relapse.

If fissures or splits occur in skin without associated callus, Steristrips can be used to oppose the edges. As in deep dermal fissures above, an emollient should be applied regularly after healing to maintain flexibility of the skin. Fissures often occur in sites where the skin is subjected to traction, and offloading of the area may help to resolve the problem.

When fissures are caught early they may not yet have extended to the dermis and remain entirely within the callus. These are managed by debriding away the plaque of callus, including the fissure in its entirety, and subsequently applying emollients regularly. Regular podiatry is important, and additional steps should be taken to prevent callus from reforming at the site by changing footwear or insoles or making a suitable orthotic.

In Scandinavia some practitioners use medical super glue to close fissures.

BURNS

The first presentation is a blister, filled with clear fluid. One of the problems of assessing the severity of burns on the diabetic foot is that lack of pain is a valuable marker of a deep burn and is absent in the diabetic foot. All large, or deep, burns should be referred to a specialist burns unit: for superficial or partial thickness burns the treatment is as for an ulcer.

SCARS

These follow ulceration or other trauma to the foot, and are very prone to break down. They are less flexible than normal tissues and are frequently associated with heavy callus formation. Scar tissue in heavy callus has a whitish rubbery appearance and is avascular. Care should be taken not to cause unnecessary trauma to the area, which may be slow to heal.

Occasionally, an inclusion cyst will develop in a scar, where epidermal cells are trapped deep in the tissues and present as a fluctuant swelling from which 'cheesy' material can be expressed. A podiatric – or other – surgeon can excise this.

MINOR AMPUTATION – DEBRIDING SURGICAL WOUNDS TO SPEED HEALING

Wounds heal from the base, where a healthy bed of granulation tissue forms, and from the edges, where new epithelium migrates across the wound. Both these processes are assisted by debridement of slough, eschar, necrosis and fibrous tissue, from the base of the wound, and by clearing the edges of callus, which can be a barrier to migration of epithelium.

REMOVING NECROSIS FROM NEUROPATHIC AND NEUROISCHAEMIC FEET

The neuropathic foot does not tolerate the presence of wet necrosis, which is a wonderful growth medium for microorganisms. As much necrosis as possible should therefore be removed by sharp debridement. In the neuropathic foot, with wet necrosis, this procedure is usually performed by a surgeon or surgical podiatrist and involves excision of all non-viable tissue.

The neuroischaemic foot is an entirely different entity. When ischaemic necrosis is wet and associated with severe infection, as much as possible of the affected tissue needs to be debrided and, if possible, angioplasty or bypass should also be performed.

However, if necrosis is dry and well demarcated, and no vascular intervention is possible which could improve perfusion of the foot, then dry necrosis is best managed conservatively. The aims are as follows:

- To debride along the demarcation line between necrosis and viable tissue, clearing the line of heaped-up debris and crusted exudates.
- To debulk non-viable tissue, which is a grand growth medium for bacteria.
- To remove necrotic tissue, which would otherwise be in direct contact with normal tissue. Interdigital areas in healthy toes adjoining necrotic toes are very vulnerable to infection and gangrene and should be separated from gangrenous areas with a dry dressing.

MANAGING EXCESSIVE BLEEDING

The surgeon who taught the author how to debride told her never to worry about bleeding unless she could hear it. All bleeding stops in the end, he added helpfully.

Before commencing debridement the operator should ascertain that the patient is not on warfarin or other blood-thinning agents. Renal patients on haemodialysis may risk bleeding if debrided on the day that they dialyse because they are heparinized while on the machine.

If bleeding occurs:

- Elevate the limb.
- Apply digital pressure to the bleeding area of the wound over a dressing for at least 3 minutes.
- If the dressing is first moistened with saline it will be easier to lift it at the end of the 3-minute period to check that bleeding has stopped, without disturbing the clot.
- Alternatively, strapping can be applied with tension over a dressing to free up the operator's hands so that she can continue working.
- If bleeding does not stop within 3 minutes, calcium alginate (Kaltostat) can be applied topically. This releases calcium ions, thus assisting the clotting mechanism.
- Podiatrists should always ensure that bleeding has ceased before the patient leaves the clinic.
- If the bleeding is heavy, advise the patient to rest and elevate the foot for 48 hours. If bleeding re-starts, another dressing should be bandaged on top of the first dressing.
- Extensive debridement should not be performed when one podiatrist is alone with a patient.

Occasionally, patients end up in accident and emergency after a podiatry treatment because of bleeding.

Case study

An 89-year-old man with type 2 diabetes of 27 years duration and neuroischaemic feet, and who was taking warfarin, had an area of necrosis on his left hallux and received regular treatment from the diabetic foot team. The area of necrosis on the apex of his left hallux became very loose and was gently debrided away by the podiatrist because it was felt that excessive motion of the necrotic area would lead to traction on adjoining tissues and possible injury. Nine hours later, the patient was taken to casualty by his family during the night because the toe had not stopped bleeding. In casualty, the bleeding stopped when the foot was elevated and a firmly bandaged dressing was applied.

Case study

A 54-year-old man with type 2 diabetes of 9 years duration, peripheral neuropathy, and extensive calcification of his pedal vessels, who walked to the bathroom without shoes in the middle of the night, knocked his ulcerated foot on the bedpost, fractured a small calcified vein in his foot and bled copiously.

DEBRIDEMENT WITH MAGGOTS (LARVA THERAPY)

This treatment has been used intermittently at least since the American Civil War. During the First World War it was observed that maggots cleaned wounds very effectively; the treatment has recently come back into fashion on both sides of the Atlantic.

The larva used are those of the green bottle fly (*Lucilia* spp.) a pretty little plump, shiny metallic green fly, the larvae of which feed on dead flesh and not on living tissues. They can therefore be used to clear away non-viable tissue and slough from wounds. They can be useful if the foot is very ischaemic with extensive slimy slough and necrosis, which is difficult to grip with forceps or cut with a scalpel.

Medical maggots are produced by medical maggot farms under stringent hygienic conditions, and other types of maggot should not be used. At the Bridgend Maggot Farm in Wales, the eggs of the flies are laid on raw sterile liver and are then collected and cleaned according to a secret formula. When the maggots hatch from the cleaned eggs they are sterile, and are delivered to clinics in a sterile clear plastic container.

At this stage they are small larvae about the length of a grain of cooked rice but not so thick. They look clean, pearly white and innocuous ('quite sweet' said one patient) and do not smell. They are rinsed out of the container with sterile saline, which is strained onto gauze to catch the maggots, which are placed in the wound, covered with a loose dressing and contained within a 'cage' made of nylon mesh, which is provided by the 'maggot farmer'. Other suppliers may provide the maggots already contained within a closed sachet.

Normal skin around the wound should be masked to prevent it becoming excoriated by the strong digestive enzymes secreted by the maggots. Some people use hydrocolloid dressings for this, but the author has always used Calorband, which can be easily lifted to inspect masked skin.

Patients undergoing larva therapy should not walk, as the maggots may be crushed or displaced from the wound interface. The foot will, anyway, benefit from pressure relief.

Over the first two or three days copious quantities of discharge, largely made up of enzymes secreted by the maggots, are produced. The exudate is a pinky brown colour. If the overlying dressings become too saturated there is a danger that the maggots will suffocate; they stand head down and bottom up in the wound and breathe through their top end (the blunter of the ends) so soaking dressings should be removed and replaced with gauze. A curious, fusty, musty odour may arise from the maggoty wound. Over the first 2 days, before they settle down to feeding, the maggots can be seen wriggling and squirming very energetically within the wound. Once they start to feed in earnest, they do not crawl around the wound so much but stay in one place with their heads down, sucking up liquefied slough and necrotic material that has been predigested by their enzymes. A group of maggots feeding side by side looks quite like a piece of honeycomb with the blunt end of each maggot representing an individual cell of the honeycomb.

On the 4th or 5th day the maggots stop feeding and start looking for somewhere to pupate. It is at this stage that they are removed from the wound. This is done by irrigating them out of the wound. The author uses a firm jet of fluid squeezed from the cut connecting tube of a litre bag of sterile water or saline. Once the maggots are out of the wound, its true dimensions and base can usually be clearly seen. If the wound was large, and very sloughy, further applications of maggots may be needed.

Spent maggots should be placed in a sealed container or tightly knotted plastic bag and safely disposed of as soon as possible, preferably by incineration.

When maggots are used on a wound that will be partly managed by other healthcare professionals, they should always be forewarned, as it is alarming to find maggots unexpectedly appearing in a wound or on a ward. The patient and family should also give consent to their use.

Sometimes, patients arrive at the clinic with foot wounds that are infested with opportunistic wild maggots. These should be irrigated out of the wound and sent for identification. The patient should be given tetanus prophylaxis and a course of antibiotics, and the wound should be observed closely for a few days.

PHYSICAL DEBRIDEMENT

Another form of physical debridement is with 'wet to dry' dressings. Plain gauze, soaked in saline, is applied to the wound bed, bandaged in place, and allowed to dry. It sticks firmly to the wound bed. When the dressing is changed the gauze is ripped off, and tissue comes away with it. This may be painful, is less precise than sharp debridement and is not recommended.

Another form of physical debridement is 'whirlpool' where the wounded foot is soaked in rapidly moving warm water, so that slough is macerated and some debris loosened. This technique is also not recommended.

ENZYMATIC DEBRIDEMENT

This consists of topical application of products containing enzymes that break down slough and necrotic material. Examples of this technique include Varidase (Wyeth), which contains streptokinase, a proteolytic and fibrinolytic enzyme, and papaya ointment, a folk remedy from the West Indies. They can lead to severe maceration and breakdown of tissues, which is difficult to distinguish from infection. Enzymatic debridement for the diabetic foot is not recommended.

ACID-BASED REMEDIES

■ Ascerbine cream (Goldshield)

This preparation contains malic acid and benzoic acid and is applied topically for desloughing and is not recommended for the diabetic foot.

There are also dangers associated with the use of ferric chloride and silver nitrate, which may cause severe tissue damage and mask infection. They are not recommended.

Corn cures are very dangerous for diabetic patients and are absolutely contraindicated.

■ Folk remedies and alternative remedies for diabetic foot ulcers

These are numerous and varied, including wading barefooted in the sea in Barbados, topical application of skin and slime from gulf catfish in Kuwait, and application of hot scrambled egg in China. They are not recommended. Laser therapy, magnets, acupuncture, marigold extracts, ginkgo biloba extract, aloe vera, manuca honey, topical insulin, and many other treatments all have their advocates but cannot be recommended until sufficiently large, properly conducted studies on their use on chronic wounds in diabetic foot patients have been reported. They are not, at present, accepted treatments in leading diabetic foot clinics throughout the world.

■ Debridement with dressings

Some dressings, such as hydrocolloids, cause breakdown of slough and can be used to debride wounds. For their action they require to be left on the wound for several days and are therefore not recommended for insensate diabetic feet because of the danger of infection or necrosis developing under the opaque dressing and not being detected until the dressing is removed. In addition, hydrocolloids render the wound bed very moist and form a brownish slimy material, both of which presentations are difficult to differentiate from severe infection with purulent discharge, and render wound assessment difficult.

Safety of dressings for diabetic feet

It is important to be aware that some woundcare products that are widely used on non-diabetic feet with protective pain sensation and a good blood supply can be inappropriate or dangerous if used on a neuropathic or neuroischaemic foot. Sometimes it is not the product itself that is intrinsically dangerous, or in any way a 'bad' product, but the fact that it may mask a problem in an insensitive foot, or prevent the patient from seeking professional advice, or might cause a problem if used in the wrong way.

Choice of specific dressings

The choice of specific dressings is a minor aspect of wound care for diabetic foot patients. It has been said that you could put almost anything on an ulcer except pressure and it would heal! Choosing one dressing over another is far less important than achieving good debridement, addressing ischaemia, relieving pressure, checking the wound regularly, and controlling infection. Instead of the common practice of choosing a different dressing when a wound is not healing, podiatrists should be exploring other important aspects of diabetic foot care, like whether offloading is effective, ensuring the vascular status is adequate for healing, making sure that the patient is following advice, diagnosing and treating infection, and ensuring regular sharp debridement of non-viable tissue, all of which, if suboptimal, are far more likely reasons for the healing failure.

The evidence base for selection of dressings

There are very many different dressings proposed for the diabetic foot, but there is no firm evidence that any one dressing is better than another for diabetic foot wounds. Many theories about wound healing and development of dressings were devised as a result of studies performed on animal models or acute wounds in healthy volunteers, and cannot always be safely extrapolated to the diabetic foot.

There seems to be no clear consensus among podiatrists or other healthcare professionals as to what is the best dressing for diabetic feet. Worldwide, the most common dressing used is probably gauze, and the most common cleaning agent is saline. Both are cheap and easily available: however, few practitioners in the United Kingdom use gauze, preferring non-adherent dressings, some of which are also quite cheap. Many ethics committees and research and development committees now question the use of gauze as a control dressing in research studies.

Many modern dressings are extremely expensive.

Controversies with choice of dressings

There is anecdotal information that in some patients with insensitive feet, deterioration of a wound under a dressing will not be detected unless the dressing is lifted frequently, and that the consequences of failure to detect infection or worsening ischaemia beneath a dressing can be disastrous. This has led some practitioners, including the author, to conclude that dressings such as hydrocolloids, which rely for their efficacy on being left on the wound for several days, may not be suitable for insensate diabetic feet. However, other practitioners such as Patrick Laing, the orthopaedic surgeon who is an expert in total contact casting, use hydrocolloids regularly under casts.

WOUNDCARE CONTROVERSIES

There are several other areas of controversy among experts when it comes to wound care and dressings.

Many vascular surgeons believe that ischaemic ulcers and areas of necrosis should be exposed to the open air and allowed to dry out and say that dressings should not be applied. Podiatrists, however, tend to feel that all wounds should be kept covered by a sterile dressing.

Some practitioners believe that alginate dressings have the capacity to plug wounds and prevent exudate from draining freely, and sometimes promote infection.

In America, and many other countries, 'saline gauze' is the standard treatment of wounds. However, in the United Kingdom, many practitioners believe that saline gauze is not a suitable treatment.

As already mentioned, opinion about the management of blisters is divided into those who open them and those who don't. Both groups are quite partisan.

'Wet to dry' and whirlpool are not recommended by many podiatrists in the United Kingdom but are widely used in the USA.

There is a school of thought that holds that diabetic foot patients should be allowed to immerse and wash their ulcerated feet when they take a bath. However, it has always been the author's practice to advise the patient to wash the foot but without including the area covered by an ulcer.

Some practitioners advocate using tap water to clean ulcers.

There is no consensus on any of the questions discussed above.

■ Cast protectors

Cast protectors are very useful for those who support non-immersion of wounds. Cast protectors are leg-shaped plastic covers which seal at the proximal end with a drawstring or sticky tape or a stretchy waterproof membrane, and are used to protect dressings and wounds while the patient is bathing or showering.

Three cast protectors which are widely available in the United Kingdom include:

- Limbo
- Xenocast
- Seal tight (Brown Medical).

Podiatrists recommend dressings for wounds for the following reasons:

- They protect the wound from physical trauma.
- They help to absorb the pressures of walking.
- They absorb exudates.
- They prevent infestation of the wound by insects.
- They prevent animals from being attracted to the wound.
- They keep the wound warm, thus stimulating healing.
- They keep the wound clean.
- Infection will be less likely.
- It can be upsetting for patients and others to have to look at open wounds or gangrene and they should therefore be kept covered.
- If the wound becomes infected, purulent discharge will be evident on the dressing and the patient is more likely to detect it.
- Dressings help to prevent and control odour from the wound.
- Dressings can be used to separate gangrenous toes from their neighbours.
- Some waterproof dressings enable the patient to bath or shower.

Ideal properties of a dressing for the diabetic foot are as follows:

- Easily lifted for regular inspection.
- Does not depend for its action on being left on the wound for several days.
- Does not render dry necrosis wet, thus increasing the risk of infection.
- 'Wicks' excessive discharge away from the wound bed and surrounding skin.
- Does not macerate surrounding tissue.
- Does not cause trauma to the wound bed when removed.
- Does not cause damage to the skin surrounding the wound.
- Does not plug the wound, thus preventing discharge of exudates.
- Does not change the colour, texture or consistency of the wound bed (thus making assessment more difficult).
- Keeps the wound warm.
- Absorbs pressure.
- Is not too bulky.
- Stands up well to the pressures of walking.
- Does not shed foreign material into the wound.

Common problems with wound care include:

- Leaving dressings on too long. This prevents regular inspection of wounds and may also lead to further associated problems, such as granulation tissue growing into the dressing.
- Applying dressings with the wrong side to the wound interface. The best dressings can be applied either side to the wound.
- Fixing dressings with over tight bandages.
- Using too much tape (this can traumatize the skin when it is removed).
- Encircling toes with tight tape.
- Not making allowances for fluctuant oedema.
- Trying to cram bulky dressings into shoes with an inadequate capacity.
- Not removing dressings and tape slowly and carefully, which can cause damage to the wound bed and tears to the skin (Fig. 8.12). Dressings that have stuck firmly to the wound bed should be soaked off.
- Not changing dressings frequently enough: after 'strike through' has occurred there is a risk of infection if the dressing is not replaced with a fresh one.
- Relying on patients to change dressings when their eyesight or manual dexterity or failure to understand what needs to be done may render this difficult (Fig. 8.13).

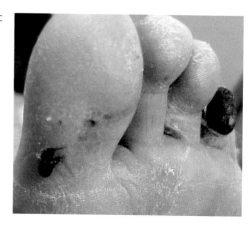

Fig. 8.12 Iatrogenic lesion caused by careless removal of tape holding dressings onto a severely ischaemic foot.

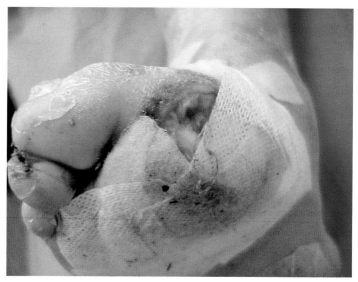

Fig. 8.13   This patient has poor vision and has stuck tape over his ulcer. Part of the ulcer has no dressing applied to it at all. Patients need careful assessment to be sure that they are capable of self-care.

In summary:

- The choice of dressings for the diabetic foot is almost infinite.
- Whatever the dressing, someone, somewhere, will be recommending it for diabetic foot ulcers.
- Choice of dressings probably makes little difference to outcomes, and there is little evidence as to their efficacy in vivo in chronic wounds of the diabetic foot.
- There is anecdotal evidence that certain dressings may mask the detection of infection, gangrene or wound deterioration in an insensate diabetic foot.
- Pharmaceutical companies are inclined to make extravagant claims about the panacea-like properties of their 'proactive' products.
- The wound care literature is riddled with pseudo-scientific papers, colour charts, case studies, anecdotes and accounts of the latest 'miracle-working' dressings for which the evidence base is worryingly thin or non-existent.

As Ali McInnis, senior lecturer at the department of podiatry of the University of Brighton and editor of the *Diabetic Foot Journal*, has often said, 'first do no harm' is the adage that should be followed whenever dressings are selected for diabetic foot ulcers.

WOUND-HEALING RESEARCH

Wound-healing research has a bad name. There are very few sufficiently large, properly conducted, randomized controlled studies, and none of them have covered wound healing in patients with diabetic feet and indolent ulceration. Two widely quoted opinions on wound care are those of Winter and Leaper. Winter published a paper in *Nature* in the 1960s reporting that acute wounds on pigs' backs healed more quickly under a moist occlusive dressing. Leaper, a surgeon working in Bristol, constructed wound care models by punching holes in the ears of rabbits and fastening a glass microscope slide cover to each side of the holes, thus constructing transparent chambers through which he could watch and monitor the growth of granulation tissue. He then removed one of the covers, applied various commonly used antiseptics, and recorded their effects on the delicate new tissue within the chambers. He saw destruction of granulations by iodine, Milton and Eusol and concluded that topical antiseptics were bad for wounds.

The work of Winter and Leaper led to profound changes in the recommendations made about wound management. However, it is easy to jump to unwarranted conclusions after reading their work and to assume that 'moist wound care' and total avoidance of topical antiseptics and hypochlorites is always a good thing. It is probably unwise to use studies on animals, or acute wounds in healthy, non-diabetic, human volunteers, as the sole basis for determining woundcare programmes for chronic wounds of the diabetic foot.

There have been several anecdotal cases of diabetic foot patients who developed infections and/or necrosis when their wounds were covered with opaque, occlusive dressings that were not changed for several days, and other cases where Kaltostat has prevented wounds from draining with subsequent severe infection.

Numerous problems are associated with designing studies to explore these areas of safety and efficacy further, because there are many different aspects to wound healing. New treatments need to be compared to accepted treatments, but there is little consensus as to what treatments are acceptable. Many studies in the past have compared new products to 'saline gauze', but many podiatrists will say that 'most things are probably better than saline gauze!'

Wound healing research is only useful if the following principles are applied:

- Groups of patients and controls should always be well matched in terms of age, sex, type, and duration of diabetes, pressure relief, blood supply to the foot, and presence and degree of infection.
- Wounds studied should be classified as neuropathic or ischaemic and stratified accordingly. It is helpful also to know the duration and size of a wound. Patients in the study should be 'stratified' on enrolment so that there will not be a predomination of large wounds or ischaemic feet or ulcers of very long duration in one group.

Above all, it is hopeless to try to measure the efficacy of a new treatment when it is being applied to dirty, infected wounds that are not being properly offloaded.

Enrolling patients for wound care studies can be slow and there is always a temptation to include as many people as possible very quickly, but it is essential first to achieve effective off-loading and infection control.

NON-HEALING ULCERS

The following are important points:

- Podiatrists should not forget the risk that the window of opportunity will close if they 'cut and come again'.
- Podiatrists should remember the time-scales for ulcer healing: after 4 weeks the podiatrist will always need help if the ulcer is not improving. The 2004 NICE guidelines for the management of the diabetic foot state that new diabetic foot ulcers should be referred to a multidisciplinary foot clinic.

When to refer immediately:

- when an ulcer is not healing within the above timescales
- if a diabetic foot becomes infected
- if a foot develops necrosis
- if ischaemia is critical (acute or chronic; see Chapter 6).

HIGH-TECH INTERVENTIONS FOR HEALING ULCERS

■ Dermagraft

Dermagraft is living human dermal tissue grown in the laboratory from cells obtained from babies' foreskins. It arrives frozen and is thawed out, cut to size, and placed on the wound bed. It is an effective treatment but extremely expensive at over £250 per application, with around eight applications needed to heal an ulcer.

■ Hyaff

Hyaluronic acid is an essential component of wound healing, and chronic wounds are often hyaluronic acid depleted. Hyaff is an ester of hyaluronic acid which is a much more stable product and remains in wounds for up to 3 days. Studies at King's showed that it is effective at closing sinuses and improved wound healing.

■ Apligraf

Apligraf is living human skin (bilayered dermis and epidermis) grown in the laboratory from babies' foreskins. It arrives in a small battery heated incubator, and is very easy to cut to size and apply to wounds. Results in achieving rapid healing of chronic neuropathic ulcers have been promising.

■ Regranex

Regranex is platelet derived growth factor grown in the laboratory from recombinant technology

   Podiatrists should understand that there is no point in even thinking about using the above advanced products on wounds unless the wound is clean and the patient will be compliant about offloading and will follow advice to the letter.

■ Vacuum-assisted wound closure

This very popular advanced technique uses a pump and suction tube to apply gentle negative pressure to the wound which promotes granulation and healing. This technique is widely used.

WOUNDCARE FOR STUMPS

Diabetic major amputees may need debridement of their stumps if callus develops on a neuropathic stump or the original amputation wound is slow to heal and accumulates debris, slough and necrosis. In these circumstances, podiatrists should be working with the multidisciplinary rehabilitation team and the limb-fitting centre.

PERCEPTIONS OF FOOT ULCERS

A patient's perception of a foot ulcer may greatly differ from that of an experienced healthcare professional. Patients might regard the ulcer as 'a little sore place' or 'a cut' or 'just a scratch'. They might regard the very word 'ulcer' as ominous and sinister, and be reluctant to accept that the 'thing' on their foot is, indeed, an ulcer. Patients may be reluctant or afraid or disgusted to look at the ulcer or take on responsibility for its care (see Chapter 9 on psychosocial aspects).

OBSESSIVE BEHAVIOUR

Some patients go to the other extreme and become obsessively interested in every aspect of their care and in seeking a cure. Patients with ulcers and their families should be discouraged from trawling the internet in a desperate search for remedies. Information on the internet can be unresearched and untried, detrimental, and sometimes downright dangerous. Patients should be advised always to discuss potential treatments with healthcare professionals before trying them out.

DANGERS OF UNDERESTIMATING WOUNDS

Healthcare professionals must always beware of underestimating the significance of diabetic foot lesions. In the United Kingdom we all work within a healthcare system that is 'symptom led'. In other words, we expect patients to complain and report their symptoms. When we are dealing with patients with neuropathy, who are symptom free and do not complain, we may make the dangerous error of believing that a pain-free wound is not as serious as a painful wound, when in fact, the reverse is often the case.

Furthermore, the reaction of GPs who are inexperienced in diabetic foot management and who might see just one or two neuropathic ulcers per year in their practice population will often differ from the reaction of a podiatrist working in a multidisciplinary diabetic foot clinic where the local diabetic foot disasters end up. It is common for GPs not to look at foot ulcers but to send the patient to the practice nurse for dressings.

ASSESSMENT OF FUTURE RISKS

After wounds have healed, most diabetic patients with previous history of ulceration should be regarded as very high risk for the development of further ulceration and need to be enrolled in a foot protection programme. The exception to this rule will be a patient who sustained a wound from a one-off acute trauma, which healed quickly without causing deformity or scarring, and who knows that he should seek help quickly if any future foot problems arise.

UNUSUAL WOUNDS

Podiatrists should be alert for wounds on the diabetic foot which do not look or behave normally. Ulcers of unusual appearance, or ulcers which do not respond to optimal care, benefit from an early dermatological opinion (Fig. 8.14).

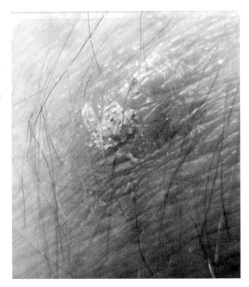

Fig. 8.14 There is more to this small lesion than meets the eye. It is a squamous cell carcinoma, which was diagnosed after being biopsied by the dermatologist.

9 Psychology and education – overcoming the barriers

He jests at scars that never felt a wound.
William Shakespeare, Romeo and Juliet II. II. I

This chapter considers psychosocial barriers to the delivery of effective diabetic foot care and the use of education as a tool to overcome these barriers.

Podiatrists working with high-risk diabetic feet frequently ask the following questions:

- Why are outcomes so poor for some diabetic foot patients?
- Why, despite education and enrolment in foot protection programmes, do some patients behave in ways that appear obviously hazardous and almost designed to lead to serious foot problems?
- How can podiatrists overcome psychological and educational barriers?

Some healthcare professionals feel extreme irritation and frustration when confronted with patients:

- whose behaviour is not conducive to good outcomes
- who do not follow advice or report problems early despite numerous problems and previous episodes of severe infection or gangrene
- who present, with gangrene, when it is too late to help them.

To understand why patients behave in these ways, it is necessary for podiatrists and other healthcare professionals to try to put themselves into the shoes of their patients and gain insight into people's motivations and the underlying causes of their behaviour before judging them too harshly.

A SHOCKING DIAGNOSIS – AND A LIFE SENTENCE

Particularly strong feelings may be aroused when diabetes is diagnosed.

● Type 1 diabetes is a disease that is difficult to forget, even for a few minutes, as it impacts on most aspects of life: working, eating, drinking, sleeping, taking exercise, going out, and almost every activity.
● The management of type 2 diabetes is very challenging, and no matter how hard patients try to control their diabetes, some will deteriorate despite their best efforts.
● Chronic illness is hard to cope with, and diabetes is a life sentence.

Illness is probably much easier to deal with if it is to be endured for a short period only and a cure is likely, neither of which is the case with diabetes. Chronic illnesses are particularly difficult to deal with because there is no end in sight. Even diabetic patients who undergo pancreatic transplantation will still remain under the care of a hospital team for the rest of their lives, even though, if the transplant is successful, they will no longer require insulin or oral hypoglycaemic agents.

Tight control of diabetes is not easy for the following reasons:

● Managing diabetes efficiently and achieving optimal blood glucose levels long term leaves little room for self-indulgence: relentless self-discipline is needed.
● Blood tests and insulin injections are unpleasant and many patients avoid frequent finger pricking and multiple daily insulin injections.
● The sensation of being hypoglycaemic is extremely unpleasant.

Patients may feel embarrassed by losing control in public if they become 'hypo' and may also be afraid of developing hypoglycaemia when they are alone or in their sleep. Because of this fear, they may be afraid to control their diabetes well enough to prevent complications in the future. (We know from the results of the diabetes control and complications trial that tight control of diabetes is associated with increased numbers of hypoglycaemic episodes.)

Patients who try to control their diabetes tightly and have frequent hypoglycaemic episodes often complain that they put on weight because of the additional carbohydrates they need to ingest to treat the 'hypos'.

Sometimes, manipulation of diabetes can be used by the patient to achieve certain desirable short-term outcomes. But patients who do this run the risk of developing severe complications. Examples include:

- Patients who use poor control of their diabetes as a mechanism for losing weight. By reducing their insulin they cannot take-up glucose.
- Patients who use their diabetes as a device to obtain increased attention from family and friends.

In short, diabetes can be a frightening, hard-to-manage, boring and tedious disease, which can never be forgotten and which makes great mental and physical demands upon patients.

Frequent reactions to a diagnosis of diabetes are:

- fear
- denial
- anger
- guilt
- bereavement
- depression
- feelings of loss of freedom
- boredom.

■ Fear of diabetes and treatments

There may be great and very real fears of future invalid status, pain, blindness, kidney failure, gangrene, amputation, and death aroused in the patient when diabetes is diagnosed or an ulcer develops. When patients attend the foot clinic they may become fearful when they see fellow patients in wheelchairs or using a white stick. Patients may worry about their future ability to earn a living, support their family and lead an active and enjoyable life. There is fear of inability to work and play.

There may be feelings of fright and physical distaste when the ulcerated foot is perceived as ugly, or smelly; and the foot can no longer be accommodated in fashionable shoes. Attractive footwear is of tremendous importance to many patients.

It takes tremendous self-discipline to follow the rules of diabetes management, and patients may be afraid that they cannot meet the demands or fulfil the healthcare professional's expectations.

In addition, there may be fear of treatment. Patients may be afraid that the podiatrist will cause an injury. When the patient has been told always to take great care of the feet it can be difficult for him to put them into the hands of a stranger who is holding sharp and gleaming instruments. It is important for patients to understand the scope of practice of the podiatrist and the reasons for specific treatments.

■ Denial of diabetes

A common human defence mechanism is to deny that a problem exists and try to put it out of the mind. Diabetes may inculcate denial. It is very easy for patients with neuropathy to:

- deny that they have a foot problem because they lack protective pain sensation
- injure their feet despite taking great care to protect them and therefore to deny that anything can be done to improve things.

Fear can lead to denial that the diabetes is a problem, or even that diabetes is present. Unfortunately, it is all too easy to forget about type 2 diabetes, which can cause few or no symptoms. It is therefore very easy for patients to enter a state of denial where they say that they 'used to have diabetes', or have 'just a touch of sugar'.

Unfortunately, some GPs, perhaps wary about alarming newly diagnosed patients, still minimize the severity of the condition and continue to disseminate fallacies about 'mild diabetes'. And so this insidious disease is poorly controlled for many years, and gives rise to problems only when it is too late to take the steps that would have delayed or prevented complications. Some patients, in addition to denying that the diabetes is a problem, will also deny ever having received education in foot care, even when this is not the case: it may be that they found the education frightening and closed their minds to it.

■ Anger

Patients frequently wonder why the diabetes happened to them and feel very strongly that it was unfair that they developed diabetes. They believe that it is hard that they developed foot problems when they were only doing what normal people do every day without thinking about it, and that too is grounds for anger and resentment. Patients feel bitter that they are the ones on whom the burden has fallen when other people who appear to neglect their health survive unscathed (Fig. 9.1).

■ Guilt

Guilt is common among recently diagnosed people with diabetes. Children may feel that they must have done something wrong for which they are being punished by having diabetes. Adults may feel that if they had watched their weight and been more active, or had a healthier lifestyle, they would not have developed diabetes. Poor management of diabetes may lead to continuing guilt and feelings of being out of control.

■ Bereavement

Patients mourn for their previous healthy status and their previous light-hearted existence when they did not need to worry about controlling their diabetes.

Fig. 9.1 The foot of an angry young man, who has never come to terms with his diabetes. He has profound neuropathy but walks barefoot around the house and presents very late.

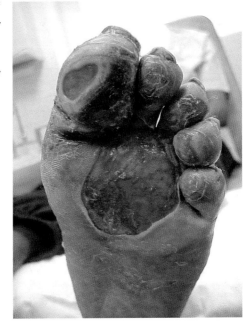

■ Depression

Depression is common among people with diabetes. Many foot ulcer patients are also depressed, and feel helpless and out of control.

■ Loss of freedom

Further strong feelings are aroused when patients develop foot problems, as these impinge upon most aspects of life. Patients with neuropathy and ischaemia can no longer take for granted the freedom to choose which shoes they want to wear, how far they can walk, and what jobs are suitable for them. When a patient develops foot ulceration the constraints on his activities, if he follows advice from the podiatrist, can become almost overwhelming. Unfortunately, however, for patients with neuropathy and ulceration, absence of symptoms and lack of protective pain make it very easy for them to deny the severity of the problem and the need to accept constraints. And, just as ignoring diabetes can lead to complications, neglect of ulcers can lead to delayed healing, severe tissue destruction, and scar formation that render relapse more likely in the future, together with infection, gangrene and amputations.

■ Boredom and the tedium of having diabetes

Diabetes is a boring disease. Continuously monitoring and balancing regimens of diet, exercise, and drugs is difficult, time consuming and dreary. Day in and day out it has to be done and cannot be forgotten.

Podiatrists should never underestimate the pure tedium for patients when, in addition to having to manage their diabetes, they also have to trek up to the diabetic foot clinic every few days, month in and month out, for a foot problem that does not hurt and may seem never to change much, and may involve:

- waiting for hospital transport to arrive
- staying at home waiting for the district nurse to call
- wearing dressings on the foot
- thinking twice about going out on impulse, accepting an invitation, going on holiday, or helping another family member or friend when this involves physical action
- worrying about how the foot will stand up to a coach trip or a walk on the sands, bathing in the sea, taking a shower, or going swimming.

Much of the joyful spontaneity of life can be lost. Diabetic foot trouble can thus have profound effects on patients, their families, and their friends.

CONCURRENT PSYCHIATRIC ILLNESS

Some diabetic patients with foot problems also have concurrent psychiatric illness, which can impinge upon their foot health. Particularly serious problems include:

- schizophrenia, which has a strong association with diabetes
- bipolar disease
- intellectual deficit.

The question to be considered is whether the patient is incapable of following important educational advice because of mental illness or intellectual deficit. If the answer is yes, then the podiatrist should ask for support from the psychiatric team (Fig. 9.2). Patients with serious mental illness usually have a personal psychiatric social worker who can be involved in decisions. Very rarely, a psychiatric patient may need to be 'sectioned' in order to deliver care for an acute foot problem.

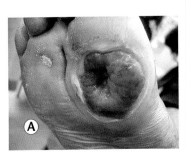
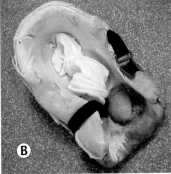

Fig. 9.2 (A) This neuropathic patient was unable to take responsibility for his foot. He would not rest. (B) A Scotchcast boot worn for 1 week by the patient whose foot is shown in (A). After being issued with the boot, he stopped keeping dressings on his foot.

The GP, the geriatric team and the social workers should also be asked to help if the patient is elderly, demented, or dangerously socially isolated.

Drug addiction leads to severe self-neglect and reluctance to accept hospital admission.

ARTIFACTUAL DISORDERS

Rarely, the podiatrist may encounter diabetic foot patients who deliberately cause ulcers and/or deliberately prevent them from healing. These patients fall under the following categories:

- Malingering: patients deliberately invent or cause illness because of the associated benefits, which may be financial or social or emotional. (The author was once asked to apply a plaster cast to the lower limb of a patient so that, when the patient appeared in court over the following days, sympathy would be elicited from judge and jury.)
- Munchausen's syndrome: sufferers fabricate signs and symptoms of illness because they enjoy being in hospital or undergoing surgery.
- Artifactual disorder: patients deliberately cause or exacerbate their problems, and often have little insight into their reasons for doing so.

All of the above cases are difficult for the podiatrist and, indeed, every member of the team, to manage. Many members of staff deeply resent being taken advantage of by these patients. However, a personal confrontation with the patient by the podiatrist is not a good idea. If confronted, the patient is likely to seek care elsewhere and their new podiatrist will not immediately understand what is going on. Patients with these disorders are seriously ill and, if discharged, self-discharged, or have their podiatric care withdrawn, they will be at greatly increased risk. Instead, they need psychiatric help and support from the entire health team.

These disorders are very difficult to diagnose and manage, and it is often only after several episodes that the podiatrist will begin to suspect that all is not as it seems. Suspicious signs include:

- unusual shape of wound
- unusual site of wound
- frequently recurring problems with no good explanation
- abnormal affect of patient.

If artifactual disorder is suspected, a case conference should be held and a decision made by the team about how best to manage the patient. Long-term outcomes are usually very bleak.

NON-COMPLIANCE

Non-compliance is not a 'politically correct' term but it usefully describes patients who persistently fail to follow advice they have received from healthcare professionals. It is important to be aware that a certain degree of non-compliance is normal behaviour in adults. As we grow up we are encouraged to:

- make our own decisions
- weigh our own judgements
- come to terms, in our own way, with the situations we have to face
- decide to what extent we are prepared to modify our behaviour.

Much is said, in this day and age, about 'patient empowerment'. However, this concept can be dangerous for diabetic foot patients, where regular professional care is necessary to manage their feet well. Some patients with complex diabetic foot problems will be very much at risk if they are so 'empowered' that they fail to follow the advice of their podiatrist. Foot problems can deteriorate with alarming rapidity and few signs and symptoms: without regular debridement, provision of suitable footwear and orthotics, and rapid control of infection, disasters can result very quickly, and it may be difficult for a lay person to make decisions about what action is needed (Fig. 9.3).

▓ Reasons for non-compliance

Patients' motives for failing to follow advice are numerous and may include many of the following:

- laziness
- boredom
- forgetfulness
- lack of comprehension
- ignorance
- lack of education
- lack of perception of the problem

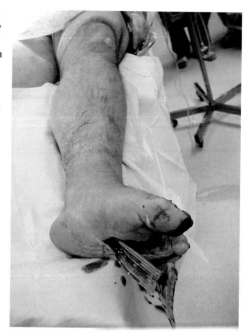

Fig. 9.3 This young man with neuropathy had a long history of neuropathic ulceration and presenting late with very severe infections. On this occasion he was toxic and shocked, with gas in the tissues, did not improve after surgical debridement and drainage, and subsequently underwent major amputation.

- too busy
- want to lead a normal life
- conflicting aims
- pressure from family or friends
- lack of money
- importance of career
- unselfishness – don't want to be a burden
- independence – 'I want to look after myself'
- denial – that diabetes, or the foot, is a problem
- desire to get on with life
- pressures of work and family life
- too hard to be a lover and an invalid
- foot problems fulfill a need for invalid status
- feelings of helplessness
- feelings of hopelessness.

LACK OF PROTECTIVE PAIN SENSATION

■ How the profound effects of neuropathy lead to '*belle indifference*'

The importance of pain is often underestimated. The message that painful stimuli are important is all pervading from birth. We are born with our own built-in alarm system that we cannot ignore. Pain teaches us to look after ourselves. We learn the 'boundaries of self' from our awareness of touch, pressure, joint position sense and pain. We know all this from the inspirational work of the late Dr Paul Brand, who worked as a medical missionary with Hansen's disease (leprosy) patients in India and the USA. Brand found that when patients lack pain sensation it is very difficult to avoid ulceration, infection, and other injuries. The miserable condition of small children with congenital inability to feel pain as a disagreeable sensation, who develop horrible injuries despite every effort to protect them, confirms Brand's views about the importance of pain as a protective and motivating force. In their vulnerability to injury, diabetic patients with peripheral neuropathy are similar to Brand's patients.

In the 'bad old days' it was not realized that tissue destruction, deformities, and autoamputations in leprosy patients were due to infections and trauma, and could be prevented. Similarly, it was believed that diabetic foot disease was due to 'small vessel disease', which could not be treated, and it was thought that diabetics who developed foot ulceration 'deserved an above knee amputation' because this would be inevitable in the end.

Unfortunately, if we lose pain we lose awareness of problems, and it is very hard to compensate for that loss of awareness. In theory we can use our brains and hands to detect the signs and symptoms of foot problems: in practice this is very difficult for patients to achieve.

NON-COMPLIANCE AND FECKLESSNESS

Podiatrists should not be too hasty to pass judgement on patients who are non-compliant. Often, all the patient is doing is behaving normally. He chooses to wear a certain pair of shoes (and peer pressure and fashion sense do not point him in the direction of podiatrically acceptable shoes for people with diabetes). He goes to work, runs for the bus, decides that he feels like taking a walk, and these simple activities lead to catastrophe … to an ulcer, to a non-healing wound, or to a Charcot foot. These simple activities are ones that the author and readers undertake every day.

Later, the patient might notice that the foot is a little swollen or pink, but it does not hurt, so he may decide on a 'wait and see' approach. These might be errors of judgement but they are not criminal offences, and patients should not be denigrated or automatically regarded as 'feckless' if they behave in these ways.

As already emphasized, podiatrists should try to put themselves in their patients' shoes … sometimes literally … and think about how they would feel if they had to wear clumpy 'granny' shoes next time they attended a wedding or important social occasion, or were banned from ever wearing a fashionable shoe or taking a long walk. They may then deepen their understanding of the patient's problems and the reasons underlying the non-compliance.

FAILURE TO KEEP APPOINTMENTS

Patients who do not attend regularly for clinic appointments are often criticized and regarded as 'feckless'. However, the burden of having to keep appointments can be very great. Many diabetic foot patients have multiple health problems and diabetic complications, which necessitate frequent hospital appointments. It is important that, wherever possible, footcare appointments are arranged to fit in with the patient's other commitments.

EDUCATION

The podiatrist's role as an educator is of paramount importance. Unless we achieve educational control, our treatments will fail. Fortunately, unlike dentists, podiatrists have patients who are able to talk back during their treatments, and much valuable information can be imparted from patient to podiatrist, and vice versa, from discussions during treatment sessions. It may be that education can overcome the barriers to effective care and early detection of problems. However, educating diabetic foot patients is not easy.

It is important for podiatrists to be aware that it is not enough to impart knowledge to patients: to keep them safe there are some other key objectives to be achieved, as follows:

- Instil the belief in patients that outcomes will be improved long term if they follow advice. Some high-risk patients may think that the damage is already done and that whatever they do, disastrous foot problems are their fate.
- Persuade patients to try and comply with the instructions they are given to the best of their ability.
- Alter the self-destructive cycle of behaviour that is common in patients with high-risk diabetic feet. Many high-risk diabetic feet belong to patients who have had trouble in the past complying with their diabetes management regimens and following advice from healthcare professionals does not come naturally to them.
- Compensate as far as possible for lack of protective pain sensation in patients with neuropathy by explaining the implications and clarifying the ways in which patients can compensate for neuropathy by actively protecting their feet, inspecting them regularly, and reporting problems early.
- Endeavour to ensure that patients believe that they are at risk but that they are not helpless.
- Teach practical preventive foot care, what is suitable foot wear, the early warning signs of foot problems, and first aid.
- Ensure that patients understand what to do and where to go when foot problems arise.
- Never regard any patient as a hopeless case.

The aim of a truly effective educator will therefore be to:

- improve knowledge
- change beliefs
- compensate for inbuilt disadvantages of lack of pain perception and tedium of coping with a chronic disease on a day-to-day basis.

To achieve these aims, it is helpful to put ourselves into our patients' shoes and begin by imagining what it is like to have diabetes. Two great educators have led the way in this field.

Dr Jean Philippe Assals, who practiced in Geneva, organized a revolutionary course for healthcare practitioners working with people with diabetes. Part of his programme involved putting course delegates into a knee prosthesis that simulated for them the difficulties of walking on an amputated limb prosthesis.

A similar approach was made by a consultant physician in Australia, who organized a special education programme for his entire diabetes team. They had to pretend that they had type 1 diabetes for a week, follow a rigid diet and record everything that they ate, take regular exercise, check their blood glucose several times a day, and inject themselves with sterile water through an insulin syringe four times a day. At the end of the week, not one delegate had been able to follow the regimen without relapsing, even though they knew that their 'diabetes' would only last for a week, and not for a lifetime, as is the case with diabetic patients.

Many podiatrists become frustrated when their attempts to persuade patients to follow advice fail. It is easy to judge patients rather harshly on occasions when they persist in wearing shoes that cause ulcers, refuse to rest, or present very late with a problem which, if caught earlier, would probably have healed quickly but which, because it was neglected, will take many weeks or months of care to heal. Podiatrists sometimes describe patients as having 'neuropathy of the brain' when they behave in this way. However, it is essential for podiatric educators to:

- Sympathize and empathize with their patients.
- Seek for the reasons why treatment sometimes fails, why patients do not accept advice, and why psychological barriers to care may prevent good outcomes.
- Imagine how they would behave themselves, if they were diagnosed diabetic or if they were asked to wear a plaster cast for 6 months, or told to refrain from walking or going to work.
- Realize that 'perfect compliance' is abnormal behaviour in adults.

Most of our high-risk patients are consenting adults. It is not natural or normal for consenting adults to follow advice to the letter, especially if the advice given:

- conflicts with their desire to lead as normal a life as possible
- opposes the wishes of themselves, their family and their friends
- marks them out as a hospital patient or stigmatizes them in some way by attaching invalid status
- prevents them from performing enjoyable hobbies or social activities
- interferes with their career or money-making capacity
- makes them feel a burden
- prevents them from wearing fashionable shoes

- is not delivered in a friendly, effective way
- is not tailored to their specific needs as an individual
- has to be followed at all times so that adherence can never be relaxed
- is not frequently repeated, explained and reinforced.

Good management of diabetes and the feet has few short-term benefits. The rewards of managing diabetes well and looking after the feet are long term and immediate rewards for 'good behaviour' are far more attractive than the promise that in years to come the patient's state of health will be improved if he follows the advice.

The advice podiatrists give to their patients should be:

- reasonable
- practical
- feasible
- relevant
- personalized
- flexible
- frequently reviewed
- regularly reinforced.

The advice given should vary in quantity, content, and method and style of delivery, depending on the individual patient's:

- age
- sex
- duration of diabetes
- occupation
- lifestyle
- complications and concurrent health problems (including classification and stage of foot)
- current behaviour
- level of knowledge of footcare, footwear and diabetic foot information
- intellectual capacity
- educational background
- psychological state
- social setting
- current stress levels.

Unless these factors are taken into account, education is likely to fail.

■ Age of patient

Young patients are often reluctant to follow advice, to wear 'sensible' shoes (trainers might be the solution), to take time off work to heal an ulcer, or to limit their social or physical activities. The young are sometimes unwilling even to agree to see a podiatrist because of a perception that only old people need podiatry.

Elderly patients might have low expectations of their health state, have difficulty coming to the clinic, and forget appointments. Some have Alzheimer's or multi-infarct dementia, which is an immense barrier to care and needs careful working with family or carers to overcome it. Eyesight may be poor and written materials should be clearly presented and in a large typeface. Sometimes it is helpful to involve a family member in education sessions.

The middle-aged or elderly male patient who lives alone and has neuropathy and poor vision is a particularly challenging patient.

■ Sex of patient

Women are frequently reluctant to wear hospital shoes. They also may not want to rest or limit their physical activity because they feel that their families need them. Mothers of young children have particular problems with achieving sufficient limitation of walking.

Men may cultivate a macho image, ignore ulcers and belittle the risks involved in non-compliance.

Diabetic foot problems affect more men than women.

■ Duration of diabetes

Newly diagnosed patients may be inundated with education from all the diabetes team and, if possible, podiatrists should not join the feeding frenzy but should stand back for a few weeks and recall the patient for education after he has had time to digest other education and begin to come to terms with his diagnosis. However, all people with diabetes should have their feet checked when first diagnosed. Type 2 patients who already have foot problems may need to be given advice or treatment immediately.

Newly diagnosed patients who are terrified of developing gangrene may need immediate reassurance.

Patients with a long duration of diabetes are more likely to have complications so the content of their education programme will need to be changed to accommodate this.

Education should be regularly repeated and reinforced; otherwise it will be forgotten.

■ Occupation

Many careers are unsuitable for patients with diabetic foot problems. Examples include:

- long-distance lorry driver
- security man, who has to continually walk around the perimeter of the site he is protecting
- porter, who must move heavy loads and stay on his feet for long periods
- factory worker standing at a machine all day.

However, once a patient is established in a career, he may feel unable to change his occupation, even if it is suboptimal so far as his feet are concerned, in which case a damage limitation exercise should be undertaken.

■ Presence of complications and concurrent health problems

The presence of these affects the content and delivery of education as follows:

- Patients with poor vision due to diabetic retinopathy find it difficult to check their feet effectively and difficult to read educational material.
- Renal complications make the feet very vulnerable to trauma and patients may be less open to education because of the pressures of managing an additional chronic illness.
- Elderly or obese patients may find it difficult to follow advice because it is hard to get down to the feet.
- Patients taking steroids will be even more prone to develop foot infections.
- Patients with history of or current ulcers, infections, gangrene or Charcot's osteoarthropathy will need additional education.

■ Lifestyle

Many patients find the constraints of a diabetic foot regimen very difficult to manage:

- Young and active patients find it hard to rest.
- Patients with a very relaxed attitude to their health may not follow an optimal diabetic regimen or detect or report foot problems early.

- Changing the lifestyle of an adult is very difficult: however, modifying it may be successful, but compromise will be necessary on the part of both patient and podiatrist.

■ Intellectual capacity

If patients have a low intellectual capacity it will be very difficult for them to understand the need for regular appointments for foot care, the need for neuropathic feet to be protected in suitable shoes, and the need to avoid danger to the feet. Often, members of the family or carers can be enrolled as informal members of the diabetic foot team who will help the patient to avoid problems.

When patients are in residential care, the staff of the home need to be educated in diabetic foot care and early detection and reporting of problems.

■ Educational background

Podiatrists should know the educational background of the patient so that this can be taken into account when delivering education:

- patient may be unable to read or write but unwilling to admit that this is the case
- very simple explanations may be needed for 'non academic' patients
- patients who are very highly educated might find it difficult to accept that they have anything to learn from the podiatrist.

■ Psychological state

- Concurrent psychological problems are great barriers to care.
- Patients with schizophrenia, severe bipolar disorder, depression, and alcoholism are prone to irregular attendances at the podiatry clinic and failure to report problems sufficiently early.
- Regular foot care will often be neglected.
- Patients who abuse drugs often have a chaotic life style and foot care is not high on the list of their priorities. Again, regular attendances and following advice are not common occurrences within this subgroup of diabetic patients.

■ Social setting

Socioeconomic factors have profound effects on delivery of care. The author works in an inner city area of great social deprivation, with many ethnic minority patients. Many patients from this background find it difficult to access care. It is important for podiatrists to gain insight into the lives of their patients and the reasons (religious, different social customs, poverty, etc.) for behaviour that is a barrier to effective treatment. Some podiatrists work abroad, and it is essential for them quickly to gain insight into the social customs and lives of their patients. For example: there are 30 million people with diabetes in India. It is customary for many Indian patients to go barefoot around the house or when they visit the temple. Thonged sandals (Fig. 9.4) are popular with patients in developing countries and lead to many interdigital lesions and traumatic injuries if the patient is neuropathic. Rat bites are common.

Poverty can lead to lack of sufficient heating or hot water, and substandard accommodation which is damp, draughty and dangerous. Patients may live high up in council tower blocks, where the lifts are unreliable and frequently vandalized. Professor John Ward from Sheffield associated poverty with increased numbers of foot problems, and the great Eliott Joslin (an early pioneer of multidisciplinary

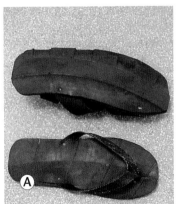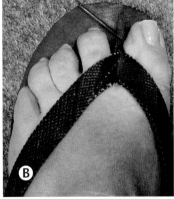

Fig. 9.4   (A) These thonged sandals are made out of car tyres and are very inexpensive and widely available in developing countries. They are held together with nails and the rubber contains metal fibres. Injuries caused by such sandals are very common. (B) A patient is wearing the sandal. The author is grateful to Dr ZG Abbas, from Dar es Salaam, Tanzania (a great supporter of the podiatry profession) for providing these footwear samples.

diabetes care in the USA) remarked that 'gangrene is a disease of poverty … it is not Heaven sent but earth born'.

■ Current stress levels

Podiatrists need to be very sensitive to their patient's current psychological state and receptiveness. Awareness of body language is a necessary skill. Leaning forward in the direction of the educator is a good sign: wandering eyes, yawns, and leaning backwards are signs that the audience is losing interest. The following points need to be taken into consideration:

● If patients are upset then it is hard for them to absorb information and follow advice.
● Patients who have suffered a bereavement have many things to do in association with the death, organizing the funeral and registering the death, and the last thing they will think of is looking after their feet.
● High stress levels make it difficult for a patient to achieve good metabolic control and hyperglycaemia may render him more susceptible to infection.
● Patients who are newly diagnosed are inundated with information from every member of the healthcare team, and it is as well for the podiatrist to stand back until things have settled down and the patient has come to terms with the diagnosis.

■ Using different techniques for imparting education and to reinforce messages

It is a good idea to reinforce educational messages when delivering education by using different techniques including:

● one-to-one sessions
● group sessions
● videos
● tapes
● quizzes
● booklets
● leaflets
● cartoons
● posters.

Sessions with 'patient educators' (patients with diabetes who are prepared to take on a teaching role and with whom the audience of patients will immediately empathize) are often helpful. Past repro-bates often make excellent educators and they avoid a 'holier than thou' effect.

For non-native English speakers, translations, and interpreters will be needed.

When preparing any educational material, podiatrists may find the following checklist useful. Is education:

- Appropriate?
- Delivered in the most effective way?
- At the right level?
- Comprehensible?
- Practical?
- Covering only the essentials?
- Is it likely to cause great conflicts?
- Is a supporting system in place? (For example, there is no point in telling patients to seek help immediately if no emergency service is available).

■ Learning by assimilation
Patients learn a lot in the waiting room and also in open-plan clinics where they can watch and hear what happens to others.

■ Using fear as a tool
Fear can be a good short-term motivator but is poor as a long-term motivator because it is a basic human protective reaction to blank out the unpleasant details or go into denial.

■ What patients need to know about diabetic feet: content of education programmes
Patients at different stages need to know different things.

Stage 1 – the low risk foot
Stage 1 patients have normal feet, but still need to know:

- that people with diabetes are prone to foot problems
- how to look after their feet
- what sort of shoes to wear
- what to do if any foot problems develop
- what care to expect (an annual review of diabetes, which includes a foot inspection, and education on diabetes management, as

good metabolic control can prevent or delay future development of diabetes complications).

Stage 2 – the high-risk foot

Stage 2 patients have high-risk feet and communicating an awareness that they are at risk is an essential component of their education. They should understand the implications of neuropathy and ischaemia and be enrolled in a trauma prevention programme, with special education on:

- How to prevent problems (including the need for regular assessments and sufficiently frequent podiatry).
- How to detect problems rapidly with a daily foot inspection (they need to know the danger signs).
- What to do and where to go when problems arise.

Many will need to be helped with their foot care because self-care of nails or calluses in patients with neuropathy, ischaemia or impaired vision can lead to disaster.

They should understand that a callus is not a trivial lesion and can lead to ulceration.

They should be told about diabetic foot problems, with descriptions of ulcers, infections, and gangrene, and discussion of the causes and methods of prevention. Use of terms like 'gangrene' should not be avoided.

Stage 3 – the ulcerated foot

Patients should understand the need for:

- multidisciplinary care (and that just going to the GP or practice nurse might not be sufficient)
- optimal offloading (with different methods of offloading being explained)
- debridement and wound care
- prevention of infection
- management of ischaemia.

Patients also need to know about ulcer care and the following aspects are important:

- how to look after ulcers
- how to keep sane with a foot ulcer

- subtle early warning signs of deterioration
- florid signs of immediate and urgent danger.

Stage 4 – the infected foot
Patients with current infection are in immediate danger and need careful education. Subjects covered should include:

- detection and control of infection
- that signs and symptoms are reduced in the presence of neuropathy and ischaemic
- why antibiotics may be prescribed, the need to adhere to regimens, and what to do if side effects develop
- why hospital admission may be necessary, and what hospital treatment may entail (intravenous antibiotics, surgery)
- signs of deterioration
- signs of improvement
- suitable dressings
- that good offloading is essential.

Stage 5 – the necrotic foot
Patients with gangrene should be admitted to hospital for assessment and management, which may involve intravenous antibiotics, drainage and debridement, and revascularization. Patients and their families need to know:

- that gangrene is not necessarily the end of the foot
- that gangrene can often be treated
- the surgical and conservative approaches to gangrene management.

If patients are subsequently discharged for conservative care, they need to understand:

- what is suitable footwear for a gangrenous foot
- signs and symptoms of deterioration and improvement
- what are suitable dressings and wound care protocols.

■ What the families and carers of people with diabetes need to know
Ideally, the families and carers of people with diabetes should be educated with the patient because the information they need will be the same. Having a supportive and well-informed spouse or friend,

who takes joint responsibility for the feet, can prevent many diabetic foot catastrophes.

■ What other healthcare professionals need to know

Doctors, surgeons, nurses, medical technicians, healthcare assistants, radiologists, psychologists, dieticians, and every member of the diabetic foot team, within hospital or community, needs to understand:

- the role of the podiatrist in diabetic foot care
- the importance of preventive foot care
- the pathogenesis of neuropathic ulcers (so they do not think that, by paring callus, podiatrists are causing ulcers)
- that diabetic foot ulcers need specialist treatment, including sharp debridement and offloading
- that infections spread rapidly in the diabetic foot and signs and symptoms can be masked or absent in the neuropathic or neuroischaemic foot.

When giving talks to other healthcare professionals, it is useful for the podiatrist to show a series of pictures of the neuropathic foot developing callus, which bleeds, blisters, and becomes an ulcer, as these pictures will give a very graphic lesson; a picture is worth a thousand words. It is helpful to show pictures of feet before and after debridement, so that the audience will clearly understand that callus is removed to disclose a pre existing ulcer, and not to cause an ulcer.

When teaching healthcare professionals how to assess, classify, and stage the diabetic foot, a patient is worth a thousand pictures: the diabetic foot comes alive when real live patients and real live problems can be seen and discussed.

Teaching care of the high-risk diabetic foot to other professionals can be achieved by organizing a special training rotation (where podiatrists, physicians, and nurses see the treatment of patients with ulcers, infections, gangrene, and Charcot feet) within the hospital high-risk diabetic foot clinic. This is also an excellent way to build strong links between hospital and community.

■ In summary

- It is quite easy to change knowledge.
- It is difficult to instil belief.
- It is hardest of all to change the behaviour of an adult.

Some of the behaviour podiatrists may wish to change is of fundamental importance to the patient: eating delicious food, following footwear fashions, etc. There will be times when it is necessary for the podiatrist just to accept what the patient wishes, and do the best she can. She must try to understand and to respect, as far as possible, the motives and desires of the patient to lead a normal life. However, when these lead to behaviour that threaten the patient's health then unequivocal advice should be given and the probable results of non-compliance should be made clear. It is often necessary to compromise. And it is essential for the podiatrist never to give up on a patient.

Case study

A 28-year-old woman with type 1 diabetes of 25 years duration (treated with diet and oral hypoglycaemic agents for the first 5 years), proliferative retinopathy, and nephropathy, had numerous hospital admissions in ketosis during her teens. When she was 18-years-old she tripped on the stairs and suffered a fracture to her left first metatarsal. This progressed to a Charcot ankle and she developed severe deformity. In her early twenties she had two hospital admissions for gangrenous toes on her right foot and underwent amputation of the 4th and 5th toes. She developed neuropathic ulcers on both feet, but frequently failed to wear dressings on her ulcers or to take antibiotics when they were prescribed, which resulted in numerous hospital admissions and meant that she was unable to find employment. Aged 28 she demanded a below-knee amputation of the deformed Charcot ankle because of the cosmetic appearance. Subsequently, she developed neuropathic ulceration of the stump, which she did not report to the rehabilitation team, preferring to stuff used household dusters into the socket of the prosthesis. It was made clear to her that most of her problems could be prevented with good footcare and regular attendance at the diabetic foot clinic but she continued to fail to present regularly or to accept care unless her foot problems were very severe. She developed end-stage renal failure and was treated with a renal transplant, but when the transplanted kidney failed after 10 years she refused further intervention and died.

10 Communications

Out of this nettle, danger,
We pluck this flower, safety.

William Shakespeare, Henry IV Part I. II. I. III

Podiatrists need to communicate well with patients, their families, other healthcare professionals, managers, and the general public in order:

- to promote the podiatry profession
- for personal career development
- to provide the best patient care
- to protect themselves.

COMMUNICATION WITH PATIENTS

Good communications with patients are essential for optimal care (Fig. 10.1). However, patients with diabetic foot complications are often very fearful people and fear can be a barrier to communication.

Stage 1 patients include the recently diagnosed, who may be confused and afraid. They may feel that they face an uncertain future with fear of the unknown, and fears of amputation, or death. Patients with foot complications fear being held back at work, not being able to work, or having to give up enjoyable recreational activities. They worry about social isolation, hospital admissions, surgery, gangrene, and blindness. Many patients with type 2 diabetes already have foot problems at the time of diagnosis. Podiatrists need to develop understanding of how illness and treatments have an impact on their patients' lives (see Chapter 9).

Patients at stage 2 and above usually know that a great deal of damage has already been done, which cannot be undone because neuropathy is irreversible, and they may feel that whatever they do the outlook will be bleak.

Patients and their relatives and friends may share similar fears and expectations. There are problems of combining the role of a lover

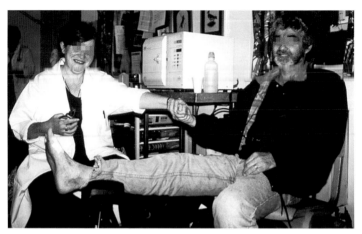

Fig. 10.1 When communicating with patients a friendly informal approach and a warm welcome are important.

and a patient, or a lover and a carer. Coping with chronic illness and the threat of amputation is difficult. Patients with current foot ulceration, and their families, often despair of ever leading a normal life again. Treatments suggested impinge on a patient's freedom. He is not allowed to choose the style of shoe he wants, he is put into plaster casts, he has to submit to regular attendances at the hospital or community clinic, he is given tablets to take, and he receives restrictions on his daily activities and admonishments for failure to follow advice.

■ Fear and anxiety as educational tools

Inculcating a little fear and anxiety can work well. Patients who have not been educated and do not realize that their feet are a severe problem may take no steps to improve the situation. Patients who are concerned about their feet, even to the extent of mild paranoia, may be more likely to check their feet regularly and seek help early. Malone, an American surgeon, educated his diabetic patients with foot problems by showing them pictures of ulcers and gangrene and found that this graphic educational technique reduced amputations significantly. However, acute or excessive fear can have negative effects, including making the patient deny the problem and the risk. Deliberately setting out to frighten patients is rarely an effective method of communicating.

Practitioners also need to be aware of the effects that fear and anxiety can have on communications with patients and their families. Patients and their families have different coping strategies and frightened people may be:

- unusually quiet
- uncommunicative
- aggressive
- loquacious.

They may forget the questions they meant to ask, and fail to take information in. It is a good idea to give the patient the direct-line telephone number of someone who can answer any questions that come to him after he has left the clinic.

Body language is an important part of communication. Friendly pats or touches can be reassuring and should be on sensate areas of the body. Eye contact should not be avoided.

A friendly, informal approach, a warm welcome and a calm atmosphere are helpful (see Fig. 10.1) The reception staff at the diabetic foot clinic should be carefully picked because vulnerable patients can be very sensitive to a brusque manner or apparent lack of sympathy.

It takes time to build relationships and develop trust.

COMMUNICATION WITH PATIENTS' FAMILIES

Communication with patients' families is very important. Clinicians need the families on their side and taking an active part in helping and supporting the patient. Families should be encouraged to accompany the patient on clinic visits. Much communication with families may be indirect. Patients and their families pick up a lot of information by talking to people in the waiting area and also by being treated in an open-plan clinic where they can observe what is happening to other patients.

People who are not native English speakers, or only understand foreign languages, need interpreters, and for practical reasons it is helpful if the interpreter is a member of the family.

It is useful for the diabetic foot team to have access to a psychiatrist if there are psychological barriers to communication.

COMMUNICATION WITH OTHER HEALTHCARE PROFESSIONALS

Effective communications with other healthcare professionals are essential. They may include:

- nurses
- doctors
- surgeons
- administrators and managers.

Podiatrists should always try to speak the same language as colleagues in other areas of healthcare, and avoid using podiatric jargon in their company which might make them feel excluded.

Podiatrists should understand that busy doctors, nurses, and surgeons will have different priorities. An overworked diabetologist might not be able to stop what he is doing and rush to the podiatry room immediately because the podiatrist wants to discuss an ulcerated foot. Diabetologists may feel unable to give foot care a higher priority than other complications of diabetes. If beds are scarce the physician may have to weigh up the merits of admitting a young type 1 patient in ketoacidosis or a type 2 patient with a stage 5 neuroischaemic foot.

Podiatrists should cultivate a confident manner but try not to be arrogant and never imply that they know a lot more than colleagues in other fields. Podiatrists should try to recognize potential jealousies and conflicts and be sensitive to the feelings of others. For example, physicians might not take it kindly if a podiatrist sends a patient to them to demand antibiotics. Many physicians worry about the cost and side effects of antibiotics and are unaware that the general principles of infection management for the diabetic foot differ from other cases. The podiatrist should always speak or write to the physician in these circumstances, explaining what is needed and why and asking the physician to consider prescribing specific antibiotics.

It is important for physicians to be educated about the role of the podiatrist. Many still regard podiatrists as toenail cutters and corn removers, and have little insight into the scope and extent of podiatric training and activities.

Nurses sometimes regard themselves as experts in wound care, largely because of their experience working with leg ulcer patients, and might need to learn that the ulcerated diabetic foot is a unique entity where the podiatrist plays an important role.

COMMUNICATING WITH MANAGERS

Podiatrists dealing with managers and administrators should be prepared to put up a sound business case for their demands. Managers in the NHS may be more concerned with providing a financially sound service than worried about the quality of health care offered. Managers need to be persuaded that podiatry is important for diabetic patients, if they are to be asked to spend money on the foot service or to pay for increased staff numbers. It is important to present them with a projection of the likely effects of any changes the podiatrist seeks to make, and the problems that may be caused if services are cut. The author has found it useful to invite managers to visit the clinic, talk to patients, and see the clinical activities.

The podiatrist should be aware of an individual manager's objectives and priorities and try help him to come up with a plan that has something positive for everybody.

When seeking funding for specific projects it is advisable for the podiatrist always to ask for more than she needs, because requests are rarely met in full.

NETWORKING

'Networking' is essential for the future of the podiatry profession. Podiatrists who work in a hospital should cultivate relationships with other healthcare professionals and administrators both within and outside the diabetic foot clinic. Podiatrists who work in the community should get to know the district and practice nurses and local physicians. Self-promotion is an important part of the podiatrist's work: she should spread the word about achievements, innovations, and successes and never turn down opportunities to meet politicians, civil servants at the Department of Health, and other people who may be in a position to support the podiatry profession and raise its profile.

COMMUNICATING WITH THE GENERAL PUBLIC

Podiatrists should avoid the use of medical jargon with laypeople and keep language simple. No opportunity should ever be missed to explain and promote the role of the podiatrist.

SPOKEN COMMUNICATIONS – GIVING TALKS

Podiatrists should welcome the opportunity to give talks, which are always an opportunity to spread the word about diabetic foot care and to promote the profession. Many people are scared of public speaking. It is a skill that rarely comes naturally and needs to be developed. However, anyone can learn to do it, and there are aids and tips that are useful in the beginning and can be discarded later with increasing experience.

■ Doing homework first

Podiatrists who are asked to give a talk should always find out how many people will be in the audience and what their background is. A talk to nurses will be different to one for doctors or patients. The most difficult audience of all is a mix of different healthcare professionals and patients together. If the members of the audience know each other and/or the speaker well then the dynamics of the group will change.

Group dynamics – the ways that a group of people will behave and respond – are curious things. Size of the group and location of the group will alter group dynamics. Although delivering a talk to a group of thirty people might not seem very different to talking to a group of three hundred people, the atmosphere will be very different, and in the larger group some of the audience will be deterred from asking questions because they are shy and inhibited by the numbers.

■ Personalizing communications

A number of 'tricks' can be used to make an audience more receptive. In these days of PowerPoint it is easy to put the date and the place on a presentation: it is a good idea to prepare a special title slide for each talk together with a slide with some local interest. If the speaker carries a laptop computer then last-minute changes to the talk can be made. Audiences warm to presenters who have clearly taken trouble and whose talks are up to date, relevant, and appear to have been specially prepared for them.

■ Attending meetings and asking questions

It is a good form of self-promotion to stand up and ask intelligent questions at meetings and podiatrists should not miss the opportunity to do this. A podiatrist who is not afraid to stand up and give her name and say that she is a podiatrist working at a particular centre is putting herself and the place she works at on the diabetic foot world map, and is also promoting her profession.

Content of talks

The subject will be predetermined but the precise content and level will need to be varied depending on the type of audience. The use of potentially disturbing clinical pictures and medical terminology should be avoided when speaking to patients or lay people.

Advance preparation for the talk includes the following:

- practising timing and presentation (before an audience of colleagues, if possible)
- asking colleagues and peers to ask difficult questions: that way, facing real questions on the day will be easier.

If a session is going to last for several hours, the audience will need plenty of breaks and the pace of the day should be varied by interspersing lectures and 'talk and chalk' with workshops (Fig. 10.2), discussions, question-and-answer sessions, and practical demonstrations. Ideally, talks should not last longer than 45 minutes without giving the audience a break or a change of style or content.

What to wear when giving a talk

Men should wear a smart suit, or trousers and jacket, with shirt and tie. There should be a pocket or belt to hold a radio microphone. Women should wear a smart suit or dress, again with a pocket or belt to hold the radio microphone. Strong plain colours work better than jazzy colours and loud patterns. Flashy jewellery distracts. If the podiatrist wears something that in itself attracts attention because it is too jazzy, untidy, informal, or otherwise unsuitable then it will distract the audience away from the speaker and the message.

Audiences are always pleased when speakers have made an effort to look smart.

Pre-talk preparations

The following pre-talk preparations are essential:

- Obtain written instructions giving full details of where the talk is to be held, including the address and the room number.

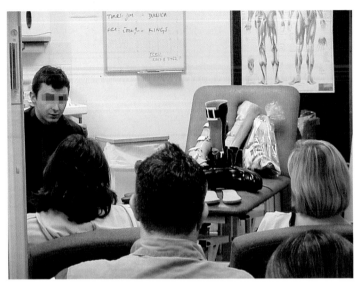

Fig. 10.2 The orthotist is holding an offloading workshop for podiatrists attending a casting course at King's College Hospital. At courses that take up a full day, a variation of pace is required, with lectures, demonstrations, practical cast manufacturing sessions and workshops interspersed.

- Clarify the type of audiovisual aids that will be available to support the talk.
- If showing clinical pictures, ensure that the venue can be 'blacked out'.
- Obtain a contact telephone number for the venue and a mobile telephone number for a contact so that if there is a problem the course organizers can be warned. Speakers should also give the course organizers a mobile telephone number.
- Speakers should arrive in plenty of time. Getting to the venue may take longer than anticipated so extra time should be allowed for this, in addition to time for assessing the venue and setting up the talk.
- On arrival at the venue, the speaker should introduce herself to the course organizer, the person chairing the session and the person in charge of audiovisual aids.

● The speaker should bring the talk on a laptop, a CD (with spare) or a flash drive, and either ask for a laser pointer to be available or bring one. If flying, the pointer should be packed in hold baggage.
● Ensure that drinking water is available and bring throat lozenges: pre-talk nervousness can make the mouth dry.

If a speaker has accepted an invitation to give a talk and subsequently has to cancel, she should offer to find an alternative speaker.

■ Audiovisual aids

A laser pointer is much better than a wooden pointer, being lighter and accurate to use. Laser pointers should not be shone on the audience!

Most speakers now use PowerPoint. As a result, the old-fashioned carousel slide projectors may not be regularly serviced and can be unreliable.

If the podiatrist is one of several speakers in a session, she should:

● sit in on the other talks
● observe the chairman's style
● watch the audience's reactions
● familiarize herself with the position of the lectern, and access to and from it.

She should seat herself in the front row on the same side as the lectern to avoid a long walk onto the platform with all eyes on her.

With experience, speakers learn to pace themselves. Nervous people usually talk faster than normal when they are giving a talk and should endeavour not to gabble, but to speak slowly and clearly. It is particularly important not to speak too quickly if members of the audience are not native English speakers.

■ Body language

With growing experience, the speaker will learn to keep an eye on the audience, considering whether they are leaning forward, and interested, or slouching back and bored or sleepy?

■ Common errors and solutions

When delivering a talk the podiatrist should try not to wave her arms or gesticulate wildly. It is a good thing to occupy one hand with the laser pointer and the other with the forward button.

A common problem with inexperienced speakers is to keep turning the head away from the microphone so that the volume of the voice fluctuates. Radio microphones should be clipped onto the side of the jacket that the head will be turning.

If written notes are used, the text should be marked with a star at points where the slide needs to be changed.

As a general rule it is good to allow for two text slides a minute, and double that number for clinical pictures.

Text slides should be kept very simple, with no more than five bulleted points on each slide.

White or yellow lettering on a dark background is easiest to read. Red and turquoise lettering is less clear.

Like extreme clothes, a very overly fancy presentation can distract the audience away from the message – keep it simple.

■ Using clinical pictures

A good picture is worth a thousand words. A series of pictures showing a course of treatment and its outcome delivers an important message. However, the quality of medical photographs that are not taken by professionals is very variable, and poor-quality pictures are far less effective.

The following points are key principles of good clinical photography which are frequently overlooked:

- the position of the foot should be standardized
- the background should be clean and tidy: large, green surgical drapes are ideal
- for a series of pictures, the view and the distance should be uniform
- lighting should be natural and avoid heavy shadows
- the patient should have given written permission and care should be taken to store images in a secure place.

■ Lecturing abroad

Podiatrists who want to be invited abroad need to cultivate the art of speaking good English very slowly and clearly and simply and remember the following:

- Invitations to lecture abroad may mean working with simultaneous interpreters: meet them beforehand, if possible, to show them your talk and discuss any potential problems.

- When talking to foreign audiences only expect to get through half the slides you would with an English audience.
- Ensure that drinking water supplied is safe to drink. (In China they often provide a flask of boiled water for the speaker: be warned that the contents may be extremely hot. The author once took a sip from a flask and blistered her mouth so badly that she had problems delivering her lecture).
- Slide projectionists in some Eastern European and developing countries are very protective of their equipment and insist on working it themselves instead of giving the speaker a remote control. They may not speak English and take a long time to understand when the next slide is wanted, which can affect the rhythm of the talk.

Speakers should be forewarned when working abroad that:

- Audiovisual aids may be unreliable.
- Power cuts are frequent in some parts of the world.
- Schedules may be exhausting.
- Requests are often made for additional lectures at very short notice, so the speaker should be able to perform without time to prepare in advance.
- It is very helpful to bring a laptop so that talks can be prepared or changed in the light of local circumstances.

Other aspects of going to speak abroad

Ascertain that speaker's expenses will be paid in full, in advance. The organizers should arrange the travel and pay for it. Speakers should never agree to pay for their own travel or hotel, even if promised a refund later, as there may be problems reclaiming it or getting the money refunded quickly.

Foreign speakers should know exactly where they will be staying or the Immigration Officers of the country they are visiting may be reluctant to admit them. The following will be needed:

- The full postal address and telephone number of where the speaker will be staying.
- The correct visa, if required. It is often possible to download forms from the embassy website to fill out in advance and check requirements and fees. Some visas are expensive and the speaker may need to queue in person at the embassy. Some visas take several days to process.
- A passport that has at least 6 months to run before expiry.

- An official letter of invitation on headed paper confirming that the speaker's expenses will be covered. Some countries also demand a letter from the speaker's employer giving permission for the speaker to go there.
- Some countries require names and contact details of referees resident in the country to be visited.
- The telephone number of a local contact is essential information.

Air travel

If the journey abroad involves taking connecting flights, it is important to be aware that some large cities have more than one airport.

Domestic airlines in developing countries may be substandard. It is best to take flights only when there is an international airport at one end of the flight.

If flights are not confirmed the seat may be lost.

Visiting speakers should always ask to be met on arrival at the airport. Even if the local language is familiar, negotiating foreign airports and finding reasonably priced transport are disconcerting, especially after a long and tiring flight.

Health in foreign parts

For some foreign venues, the health implications of staying there should be checked, and in particular:

- What immunizations are essential or advisable.
- Whether malaria prophylaxis is necessary (this varies, depending on areas within countries and local strains of the disease, and needs to be started before the trip begins).
- What other special precautions need to be taken (including drinking and cleaning teeth in bottled water only, and avoiding ice cream, salads and 'street food'). The internet is a useful resource for checking on these aspects of a trip.

■ Fear of public speaking – notes for nervous speakers

Like most novel aspects of life, public speaking becomes more pleasurable with experience. Few things impress colleagues, bosses, and potential employers more than the ability to deliver an excellent talk in a confident manner. Public speaking can raise money for the podiatry department. After delivering a talk that goes well there is a feeling of joy and achievement.

Most people are nervous and inexperienced in the beginning. It may be useful to:

- read from a double-spaced script
- write the key points down on flash cards
- get a page printout of the PowerPoint text slides and cut them up to make a little (stapled together) booklet, which can be held in the palm and used as a crib sheet if necessary.

■ Handouts

Handouts and a short speaker's curriculum vitae should be prepared well in advance. However, handing over an exact printout of every slide risks future plagiarism. Speakers and writers should be aware that once pictures have been published then, even if the author and publisher officially retain copyright, they have lost control of the images, which may appear in other people's talks.

A few new pictures and fresh text slides should be included every time a talk is given: each talk should be unique.

It is well worth doing a PowerPoint course, buying a decent digital camera, and taking pictures regularly in clinic.

CHAIRING MEETINGS

The role of chairman includes ensuring that the audience and the speakers feel comfortable, enjoy themselves and gain something from being there, and that speakers keep to time.

The chairman should always be sure to prepare questions in advance for any speaker in the session being chaired. Every speaker deserves a question and if none come from the audience then the chairman should step in. The chairman's question will often lead to more questions from the audience. The chairman should also start off applause at appropriate moments and thank the speakers and the sponsors.

Nothing kills the atmosphere of a meeting more quickly than not allowing speakers to take questions immediately after their talk has finished. It is sometimes the custom to save up all questions for individual speakers for a panel at the end of the session where all the speakers sit up in front, but this approach makes a meeting very flat. Taking questions immediately after talks does not preclude holding a panel session later.

Meetings are an invaluable way for podiatrists to get themselves known and build their careers. At job interviews a serious candidate will be expected to talk about conferences she has attended and participated in.

COMMITTEES

Sitting on committees can be alarming, especially in the beginning, or if the podiatrist is invited to join a committee late in the day, after the other members are used to working together. It sometimes seems as if everybody else in the committee is an eminent physician or a member of a clique. Committees are invaluable for networking but pressure needs to be put on organizers of meetings not to hold them in prime clinical time.

DEALING WITH THE MEDIA

Different Trusts have different rules for their employees. It is generally unwise for a podiatrist to speak to journalists about any aspect of her work without first seeking guidance from the Trust's Department of Corporate Communications.

WRITTEN COMMUNICATIONS

■ Writing papers

The literature of podiatry is alarmingly sparse. For the profession to grow and thrive it is essential for podiatrists to write more papers and books.

As a matter of courtesy the podiatrist should discuss any proposed papers with close colleagues and, if they have played a part in the work, this should always be acknowledged in papers. Podiatrists must never take undue credit for other people's work or knowingly plagiarise.

When allocating credit it is better to be over generous than to be mean; however, people should never be given false credit for work they have not done, as that is intellectual fraud. It is unfortunate when workers from different centres appear to have an arrangement that author names from both centres will automatically appear on any paper from either centre. The lines between giving advice and actively participating in the work done may need clarification.

Before the podiatrist starts to write a paper she should always:

● conduct a literature search to find other relevant material on the same subject
● decide at which journal the paper should be aimed
● refer to specific author's guidelines, many of which can be downloaded from a journal's website
● read back issues: many papers need tailoring to fit an individual journal's house style.

Most journal editors are delighted to discuss proposals for papers and offer helpful comments early on in the process.

Papers should be submitted to reputable, peer-reviewed journals. Podiatrists from the United Kingdom may find it easier to get a paper into a British journal than an American one. Journals interested in papers on the diabetic foot include:

● *Diabetes Care*.
● *Diabetic Foot Journal*
● *Diabetic Medicine*
● *Journal of the American Podiatric Medical Association*
● *Journal of Podiatric Medicine*
● *Journal of Wound Care*
● *Podiatry Now*
● *Practical Diabetes International*
● *Nursing Standard*
● *Nursing Times*
● *The Foot*

Of the above journals, *Diabetes Care* and *Diabetic Medicine* are the most prestigious.

■ Joining organizations

Organizations with an interest in the diabetic foot who hold regular meetings include:

● Diabetes UK
● The South East Thames Regional Health Authority (SETRHA) Diabetic Podiatry Group
● The Diabetic Foot Forum
● The United Kingdom Society of Chiropodists and Podiatrists
● The European Association for the Study of Diabetes (Postgraduate Diabetic Foot Group)

- The International Diabetes Federation
- The American Diabetes Association
- PDUK, Diabetes UK's Diabetic Foot Group

The reasons for joining diabetic foot organizations include:

- meeting other people working in the same field
- meeting like-minded people and fellow enthusiasts
- avoiding isolation and keeping up to date
- having an opportunity to present work.

Many organizations hold regular meetings where clinical and research work can be presented. An abstract needs to be submitted (usually around 200 words). Details of meetings, rules, and deadlines for abstract submission can usually be downloaded from an organization's website. It is helpful to obtain books of previous abstracts to get a feel for the language, style, and construction of previously successful abstracts. Abstracts can be considered for oral or combined oral and poster. Oral presentations have far more prestige and do not preclude the work being accepted in poster form. Having an abstract accepted is a great honour and employers or pharmaceutical companies will usually be prepared to assist with attendance expenses.

■ Writing book chapters

Podiatrists who have gained experience in the field of diabetic footcare may be asked to contribute a book chapter to a volume edited by someone else. The following information will be needed before writing starts:

- proposed area to be covered
- list of other authors and the content of their chapters to avoid repetition
- number of words
- number of pictures (colour or black and white)
- number of tables
- style
- footnotes
- delivery date.

The author should keep to the deadline set by the editor, and keep in touch with him, raising any problems as soon as they develop.

■ Writing books

Podiatrists should not begin writing a book until they have a publisher's commission and a signed contract; otherwise they may be wasting their time. However, podiatrists do not have to wait to be approached by an interested publisher: instead they can contact publishers with a proposal. Most publishers have websites giving information to prospective authors. When submitting a proposal it is important to be clear about:

- proposed content
- proposed format (size, length, the number of illustrations and tables)
- the likely audience
- what is new and attractive about the proposed book
- existing competition.

Writing a book takes up valuable spare time – both evenings and weekends – collating and writing. Prospective authors should multiply the anticipated workload at least ten-fold to get a realistic idea of the commitment needed. Writing is lonely, hard, and painful, but the satisfaction is great. In the world of books, the profession of podiatry is grossly underrepresented, and there is a great shortage of good podiatry textbooks.

■ Ghost writing

Podiatrists should always be extremely wary about appending their name to something that has been written by someone else, particularly if that someone else is working for a pharmaceutical company.

■ Organizing material for a book

A good-quality flash drive is beyond price.

- the flash drive should only be used for the book.
- material should be backed up every day without fail, preferably on more than one computer.

This sounds paranoid but is essential. Like humans, computers can die suddenly or be stolen away.

If the author cannot keep to a deadline, the publisher's editor should be told as early as possible that there is a problem keeping to time.

LITIGATION AND THE DIABETIC FOOT

■ Good communication can prevent litigation

In the twenty-first century, podiatrists are working within a litigious society. It is important to be aware of the need for caution when managing the diabetic foot, because this is a field where things can go wrong with alarming rapidity and sometimes for no obvious reason. This is very disconcerting to the patient, who may seek a scapegoat if his foot suddenly turns black and comes to amputation and he was not forewarned that this might happen and does not understand the reasons why the foot went so wrong.

Case study

A 54-year-old woman with type 2 diabetes of 20 years duration and neuroischaemic feet, developed painful plaques of thin glassy callus over her metatarsal heads. She attended the diabetic foot clinic, her callus was debrided, and a small haemorrhage occurred. The area was cleansed with normal saline and dressed with a sterile non-adherent dressing. The pressure index was measured: it was 0.7. The patient was asked to re-attend for a check in a week's time and was carefully educated in detection of problems and the need for daily inspection of the foot. She did not attend in 1 week and, when her home was telephoned, the clinic staff were informed that she had gone on holiday to Canada. She returned to the clinic 6 weeks later, with a large infected ulcer on the site of the previous haemorrhage, and said that she intended to sue the podiatrist who had cut her foot. She was admitted to hospital and given intravenous antibiotics. An angioplasty was performed to improve perfusion of the foot and the ulcer healed in 4 months. It was pointed out to her by the diabetic consultant physician that had she followed the advice she had been given, and kept her appointment, it is likely that the problem would have been controlled much earlier. The patient's notes had been properly filled in, recording the 'haem' together with the advice given, and signed and dated. The patient decided not to sue the podiatrist.

The likelihood of litigation can be reduced if patients and other healthcare professions are well informed about:

- the full scope of practice of the podiatrist
- reasons for interventions
- possible problems that might arise.

All diabetic patients with foot problems should be taught the:

- natural history of the diabetic foot
- pathogenesis of foot ulceration, Charcot's osteoarthropathy, infection, and gangrene.

If patients and their families understand the reasons why foot problems have developed and the reasons why the foot has deteriorated, they may be less likely to hold the podiatrist responsible.

It is human nature to blame the last person who saw the foot before problems arose for having caused the problems. The podiatrist will frequently be the last person who saw and treated the patient before the problem developed, and is therefore particularly liable to be blamed.

It is important for the podiatrist always to try to put herself into the patient's shoes and realize how disconcerting it is when a stranger in a white coat takes up a scalpel and makes the foot bleed, or when at an apparently routine visit to a podiatrist, callus is pared, and the podiatrist then announces that the foot is ulcerated. Patients are very liable to link cause and effect erroneously and suspect that it was in fact the podiatrist who carelessly cut the foot and caused the ulcer. Podiatrists are always at risk of being falsely accused if they remove callus to reveal an ulcer of which the patient was previously unaware: 'I went to that chiropodist who cut me while taking off hard skin and caused the ulcer' is a story we have all heard.

Performing vigorous debridement of a neuropathic ulcer in an inexperienced patient, which leads to bleeding, can upset both patient and other healthcare professionals who are not aware of the benefits of debriding the ulcerated but well-perfused neuropathic foot. The author once read an expert opinion from an eminent consultant physician who wrote that 'chiropodists should never cut or stretch the flesh of a diabetic foot.'

Further problems can arise if a patient develops an infection or gangrene and a podiatrist was the last person who treated the foot. Accusations may be made that the care was negligent and led to the problem.

Scenarios like the above are alarmingly common and can lead to podiatrists being reported to the Health Professions Council for negligence or being made to appear before local committees of enquiry. All practising podiatrists should realize that they are vulnerable and should take active steps to protect themselves from false accusations of negligence. Protective steps include the following:

- The notes: these should be written in black ink, signed and dated, and retained for at least 7 years after the treatment episode. They should contain details of treatment delivered and treatment refused. For all diabetic patients the presence of neuropathy and ischaemia should be recorded and if the foot is high risk, then details of education, footwear and offloading should be noted.
- The diary: this should be a precise record of when, where and by whom patients are seen.
- Being sensitive to the special needs of patients: high-risk patients in trouble should have short appointment intervals and be advised to return early if problems arise.
- Chasing missed appointments: if high-risk patients miss an appointment they should be telephoned and sent another appointment. If they fail to attend again, the GP should be notified. If the patient is very frail it may be necessary to check whether they have been taken ill at home.
- Contacting the GP: if patients do not follow advice, or any aspect of their care gives rise for concern, the concerns should be set down in writing and sent to the GP or diabetic clinic: a copy should always be retained for the podiatry notes. If the GP is telephoned this should be recorded in the notes. If high-risk patients ask to be seen between their regular appointments they should not be turned away.

RELATIONSHIPS WITH PATIENTS AND THEIR FAMILIES

It is sometimes said that patients should never be regarded as friends. The author has mixed feelings about this statement. If a podiatrist sees a patient every week or two for many years and gets to know them very well then the fine line between patient and friend may become blurred. Becoming emotionally involved with patients is a bad thing if it affects care; however, there is room for friendship and affection, especially after many years of caring for a patient, so long as these emotions do not affect the sound judgement of the clinician and so long as there is no favouritism.

■ When patients die

Part of the role of the podiatrist may involve seeing and comforting relatives after a patient has died.

It is probably unwise to go to a patient's funeral without a specific invitation: some families like to grieve in privacy and death arouses strong emotions, some of which may be directed against those who cared for the patient but could not prevent him from dying. However, if a podiatrist is specifically invited to a funeral then it is a good thing for her to go, if she can. By doing this she will be supporting the loved ones of her patient, and the cathartic effect can be helpful and consoling for the podiatrist as well as the family. Podiatrists who specialize in the care of high-risk diabetic foot patients will see many of them die, which is upsetting, especially if they have known the patient for many years.

Letters of condolence should be sent to the families. Some patients' relatives like to come back to the clinic, talk to staff and thank them, and often offer wheelchairs and walking aids for the use of other patients.

Some families want explanations about what went wrong and why the patient died or lost a leg. The podiatrist should see them together with the physician to explain what happened.

The podiatrist should sign-off the notes formally with the place of death, date of death, and cause of death, followed by 'rest in peace'.

■ When things go wrong

Podiatrists may be accused of sins of commission and sins of omission if a patient deteriorates, gets gangrene, undergoes an amputation or dies. The podiatrist may be accused of causing problems by:

- failing to assess the foot properly
- making the wrong diagnosis
- failing to see or review the foot sufficiently frequently
- failing to provide adequate treatment
- failing to refer onwards in a timely fashion
- failing to provide offloading
- failing to educate the patient
- failing to warn the patient of possible outcomes.

They may be accused of damaging the patient by:

- causing an injury (accidentally cutting the patient or removing too much callus)
- causing an infection
- causing gangrene
- causing amputation
- causing pain and disability.

All practising podiatrists should take out insurance to cover them against claims of injury or negligence.

The podiatrist's duty of care is to the patient but she also has a duty of care to her employer and should follow local Trust guidelines.

If a podiatrist feels that a patient has been put at risk or damaged by the action or omission of a podiatrist or other healthcare professional, then she has a duty to speak out, although this may be morally very difficult. In these circumstances, most Trusts ask for a form to be filled in and handed to managers if a patient's well-being has been jeopardized. However, in most circumstances it is not helpful to criticize colleagues or other healthcare professionals, or the care previously offered, too vehemently. 'There but for the grace of God go I' is an adage to be remembered always.

■ Enquiries and Court appearances

HPC-registered podiatrists may be called on to attend an enquiry, a disciplinary hearing or a court for the following reasons:

- as a defendant
- as named 'friend' of a defendant
- as a witness
- as a manager, to present the case for or against the defendant
- to sit on a committee that is hearing a case.

Court appearances

Courts are very frightening to the inexperienced and to those on the receiving end of justice. Pomp and pomposity are often disconcerting to the uninitiated. When in court, the key points to remember are:

- The podiatrist should always talk directly to the judge and address all statements, including answers to a barrister's questions, to the judge.
- Be polite.

- Avoid jargon and medical terminology.
- The podiatrist should not be afraid to:
  - stop and think about what she is going to say
  - say that she does not understand a question or to ask for a question to be repeated or explained
  - say that she does not know the answer to a question.

WHAT TO DO WHEN A MISTAKE HAS BEEN MADE

The podiatrist should try to limit the damage by rectifying the mistake as quickly as possible. By doing this, harm to the patient may be prevented. The event should be recorded, and if harm has occurred a manager should be informed.

It may be wise for the practitioner to contact the Society of Chiropodists and Podiatrists or other professional body and seek early advice from their legal department. Podiatrists should be cautious about self incrimination.

Case study

Many years ago the author referred a female patient for nail surgery to a chronic onychocryptosis, which had failed to resolve with conservative care. The patient had no neuropathy and no ischaemia. A local Chief III podiatrist, largely involved in management, had decided that he needed to update his clinical skills and joined the nail surgery team treating the patient. He was working with a newly qualified colleague and a foot care assistant. He injected local anaesthetic, applied a tourniquet to the third toe, and removed the nail, topping up the local anaesthetic when the patient complained of severe pain during the procedure. It was only after the patient commented that she had not expected him to operate on her third toe that he realized that the offending cryptosis was on the second toe, which was the toe that he had anaesthetized. He had operated on the wrong toe. He then removed the second toenail as well, and made no mention of his error in the operation notes. His junior colleague reported him to their manager and after an enquiry he received a written warning.

Podiatrists should never be tempted to change what they have written in the notes, or make a false entry but should always remember that:

● case notes are legal records
● changing the legal record is a criminal offence.

It is very easy for forensic scientists to detect that changes have been made to notes or additions have been made at a different time to the original entry.

Self-protection

The podiatrist's protective feelers should always be out. She should be sensitive to subtle nuances of human behaviour. If she senses that she might be accused of wrong practice then it is a good idea to record, sign and date a witnessed account of what happened as soon as possible. Such an account, *made before any accusations or charges are laid*, can be very useful.

The podiatrist should make full notes, of what was said and done by whom, and attach them to the patient's records.

When patients complain it is usually because they have a profound sense of grievance: that people have treated them badly, did not tell them what was going on, did not explain the reasons for the treatments offered or did not warn them when things were going wrong. Sometimes this is due to poor communications. Litigation is more likely if the podiatrist:

● is perceived as being nasty, unkind, lazy, rude, incompetent, or arrogant
● has failed to build friendly relationships with patients and other healthcare professionals
● does not bother to explain what she is doing and why it is necessary
● does not forewarn patients
● does not apologize or explain when things go wrong
● does not keep good records.

Being an expert witness

Podiatrists with extensive experience in the field of the diabetic foot may be asked to act as expert witnesses.

Writing reports

Initially, the work of an expert witness will involve preparing a report on what happened. The podiatrist should charge a realistic amount for this. At the time of publication, the going rate is around £80 per hour for preparing and writing a podiatry expert witness report.

Layout of the report

The expert witness should say who she is, what her qualifications are, what her position is, what papers relating to the case she has had access to, and whether she has examined or interviewed the plaintiff or spoken to anyone else involved with the case.

She should always remember that she is preparing the report for the court, and not for the solicitor who briefs her or his client. The expert witness's duty is to the court and to the court alone.

She should never lie and never exaggerate. Before she makes sweeping criticisms she should remember that the duty of care of the podiatrist is to act in a reasonable manner, and perfection cannot be expected all the time. Inexperienced community podiatrists should be safe practitioners but they do not have to be specialists.

Sometimes the court will dictate that the expert witness must meet the expert witness(es) for the opposing side to see what aspects of the case can be agreed.

Sending in the bill

The expert witness should quantitate and cost her activities: so many hours for preparing the report, so many hours writing the report, postal charges, telephone calls, and other expenses. The bill, on headed paper, should request payment within 1 month, making it clear that compound interest will be charged if the bill is not paid, and monthly reminders should be sent. Some firms of solicitors are extremely tardy about paying bills. The expert witness will need to keep records of her private work for the taxman.

None of the papers relating to the case should be destroyed. They should be returned to the commissioning solicitor when the case is completed.

▉ Acting as a visiting expert

Podiatrists may be asked to comment on footcare services, highlighting problems and proposing solutions.

Data may be gathered from previously published reports and documents, from interviews, from field trips, from confidential requests for information, and from government White Papers.

ORGANIZING COURSES

There is a great demand for podiatric education and podiatrists may wish to organize courses, both 'in house' and for healthcare professionals from other Trusts.

The major costs involve hiring a venue with suitable seating and audiovisual facilities, organising catering and advertising the event.

When organizing small courses at King's, our main clinic room doubled up as a teaching room. We projected directly onto a white wall at one end of the clinic and by using lightweight stacking chairs we could seat 50 participants. Our reception area, with a big round table, doubled as the catering area where tea, coffee, and a curry lunch catering for both carnivores and vegetarians, obtained from a small, local, family firm, was laid out.

Delegates were asked to pay for the course in advance and not allowed to attend if funding had not been received.

We never advertised the courses in journals: instead, advertising flyers were produced and when members of the department gave talks or attended other conferences then delegates were told about the course.

Sponsorship and free samples for practical workshops were obtained from pharmaceutical companies.

In this way, everything was kept under one roof and under the control of the conference organiser, costs were minimal, and valuable funding was obtained for the diabetic foot clinic.

11 New roles for podiatrists

Perceptions of the podiatry profession

There is a tide in the affairs of men,
Which, taken at the flood, leads on to fortune;
Omitted, all the voyage of their life,
Is bound in shallows and in miseries.
On such a full sea are we now afloat,
And we must take the current when it serves,
Or lose our ventures …

William Shakespeare, Julius Caesar IV. III. 217

To many uninformed people, podiatrists are still the 'base corn cutters, sow gelders' described by John Marston in the seventeenth century, and it is important to change and improve public perceptions of our profession.

One of the advantages of the modern term – podiatrist – over the old-fashioned term – chiropodist – is that many members of the general public will ask what it means. It thus gives podiatrists a chance to explain their role without being prejudged as a 'toenail cutter'.

Podiatrists should never miss out on opportunities to talk to and work with healthcare workers from other professions, even if members of other professions are condescending at first.

It is very important for podiatrists to try to combat ignorance and patronage. This should be done preferably in a charming and non-confrontational way, teaching by example.

BREAKING DOWN INTERPROFESSIONAL BARRIERS BY WORKING WITHIN MULTIDISCIPLINARY TEAMS

Traditionally, podiatrists in the United Kingdom have worked in isolation but it is now more and more common for the podiatrist to be a member of a multidisciplinary healthcare team. It is easier for other healthcare professionals to absorb information about our roles and competencies if they can do this by having the opportunity to work alongside us.

Different multidisciplinary teams can include podiatrists, and the list of different teams is rapidly growing as podiatrists take on fresh challenges and develop their careers without having to surmount some of the barriers encountered by previous generations. Different multidisciplinary teams dealing with the diabetic foot (not necessarily exclusively) include:

- The community multidisciplinary team: podiatrist, general practitioner, practice nurse, district nurse. These groups are likely to play an increasingly important role since current policy in the United Kingdom NHS appears to be that diabetes should be managed in the community wherever possible.
- The hospital multidisciplinary diabetic foot team: podiatrist, diabetic physician, diabetes specialist nurse, orthotist, surgeon, radiologist, microbiologist. This model is the only one which has been shown to be effective in reducing major amputations in people with diabetes.
- The rehabilitation team: rehabilitation specialist physician, physiotherapist, occupational therapist, orthotist, prosthetist and podiatrist.
- The renal team: renal physician, surgeon, nurse, podiatrist.

The role of the podiatrist within the multidisciplinary team includes:

- Working in joint clinics with other team members to diagnose problems and plan and deliver treatments.
- Offering regular, sufficiently frequent, preventive footcare.
- Wound care including sharp debridement for ulcer patients and selection of dressings.
- Footwear advice and modification.
- Ordering, manufacture and provision of orthotic devices and liaising with the orthotist.
- Advanced offloading techniques including total contact cast and Scotchcast boot.
- Educating patients, their families and carers, and other members of the multidisciplinary foot team.
- Manning the emergency service to provide same day access for high risk patients in trouble.

Some of this work will take place in joint clinics.

▓ Definition of a joint clinic

A joint clinic is a clinic where different healthcare professionals regularly work together within the same clinic room at the same time. A podiatry room appended to a diabetes centre, where the podiatrist works alone, occasionally seeking help, is not a joint foot clinic.

SPECIALIZED ROLES

Specialized roles for podiatrists within the field of diabetic foot care include:

- the diabetic foot practitioner
- the consultant podiatrist
- the podiatric surgeon
- the transplant podiatrist
- the rehabilitation podiatrist
- the research podiatrist
- the podiatrist who is working abroad
- the expert witness.

▓ The diabetic foot practitioner

Hospitals are now beginning to appoint podiatrists to a novel role: that of the diabetic foot practitioner. This ground-breaking role helps to lower some of the barriers between the roles of podiatrist, nurse, and physician, and ensures continuity of care between inpatients and outpatients with diabetic foot problems. The diabetic foot practitioner is based on the ward, with responsibility for organizing care for diabetic patients who are admitted to hospital with foot problems. She:

- liaises with and works with other members of the multidisciplinary team on the ward
- inspects the feet of inpatients on a daily basis for signs of deterioration and improvement
- performs frequent sharp debridements
- manufactures pressure relieving devices (Fig. 11.1)
- books angiograms and other investigations
- ensures that appropriate medication is administered promptly
- organises pressure relieving mattresses to prevent pressure ulcers
- ensures that treatment regimens are followed

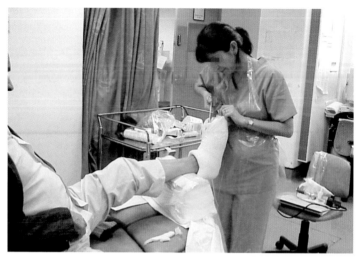

Fig. 11.1 The diabetic foot practitioner has come down from the ward with a patient to fit a Scotchcast boot.

- checks blood and microbiology results
- attends ward rounds, case conferences and angiology meetings
- alerts the team when problems develop
- educates nurses and junior doctors on the wards.

When the time for discharge arrives, the diabetic foot practitioner organizes follow-up care in the patient's home and in outpatient clinics, booking appointments as appropriate.

The role of the diabetic foot practitioner is extremely demanding. New posts cutting across interprofessional barriers are often stressful and tiring, and the place within an appropriate team of a new post is not always immediately clear to everybody – including the new practitioner!

■ The consultant podiatrist

The consultant podiatrist can play a key role in organizing the diabetic foot service. Most consultant podiatrists in the National Health Service have postgraduate surgical training and some have had training in the USA.

Consultant posts are usually broken down as follows:

- 50% clinical
- 25% teaching and advising
- 25% research.

There are a number of consultant podiatrists with a great interest in the diabetic foot. Some can offer, in addition to the roles previously discussed above:

- surgical treatment of ulcerated or infected feet
- prophylactic surgery to prevent ulcers, including osteotomies, exostectomies, etc.
- prescription of antibiotics under patient group directives (see below).

Group directives

To set up group directives relating to antibiotics for the diabetic foot it is necessary for the podiatrist to work together with the consultant physician and the department of microbiology to agree guidelines and treatment protocols.

One of the first consultant podiatrists to take on prescribing rights under patient group directives was Frank Webb, from Salford Royal Infirmary. He has always emphasized that improved prescribing rights imply increased responsibilities, and that prescribing antibiotics for high-risk patients, who are often taking numerous other drugs and may have renal impairment, is very complicated, and cannot be undertaken lightly.

■ The foot surgeon

Surgery performed for diabetic foot problems by podiatrists includes elective, prophylactic, emergent and emergency procedures.

Procedures performed by podiatrists trained in surgery can include:

- incision and drainage of infection
- proximal interphalangeal joint arthroplasty for rigid hammer toe deformity
- distal interphalangeal joint arthroplasty for rigid mallet toe deformity
- hallux interphalangeal joint arthroplasty for hallux rigidus
- Keller's resectional arthroplasty for indolent PPL ulceration
- sesamoidectomy

- lesser metatarsal osteotomy
- Weil osteotomy
- metatarsal head resection
- Achilles tendon lengthening
- partial calcanectomy
- digital amputation
- hallux amputation
- Faraboeuf amputation
- ray amputation
- transmetatarsal amputation
- midfoot amputation
- Lisfranc amputation
- Chopart amputation
- Symes amputation.

Surgical procedures for the Charcot foot
These include:

- exostectomy
- open reduction and internal fixation
- tibeocalcaneal fusion
- bone grafting
- intramedullary nailing.

The results achieved by podiatrists performing surgery usually compare well with results from orthopaedic surgeons. Some orthopaedic surgeons who are not interested in the diabetic foot may delegate foot procedures to inexperienced junior staff, who work without adequate supervision and achieve poor results.

Training to become a podiatric surgeon is long and arduous.

■ The transplant podiatrist
The transplant podiatrist specializes in the management of the feet of patients who have undergone transplantation of the kidney, pancreas, or liver. Diabetic patients who have undergone a transplant are very high risk. However, with good foot care, education, and regular inspections it is possible to reduce major amputations and gangrene.

■ The rehabilitation podiatrist
The rehabilitation podiatrist works within the rehabilitation team, managing patients who have undergone a major amputation, a high

proportion of whom will have diabetes. The remaining foot of major amputees is at great risk of developing problems: morbidity and mortality associated with diabetic major amputation is very high and within 3 years, half of the patients will be dead, and of the survivors, half will have lost the other limb. However, as with most diabetic foot trouble, regular podiatry as part of a multidisciplinary team approach can reduce morbidity.

▓ The research podiatrist

Podiatrists can play an important role as researchers. As a profession we often underestimate our worth, and some pharmaceutical companies try to take advantage of podiatrists by asking them to gather data or test products without proper support or payment. Podiatrists should never agree to do unpaid research or gather data for nothing, or in return for free samples of products (except if they are performing informal pilot studies on very small groups of patients). Mere provision of dressings or other products is insufficient recompense. Properly conducted research is a valuable commodity.

The role of the research podiatrist includes:

- making applications for grants
- helping to develop drug study protocols
- obtaining ethical committee and research and development committee approval for studies
- selecting and enrolling suitable patients according to inclusion and exclusion criteria
- organising appointments and following up patients
- working within ethical and financial constraints
- gathering data and filling in forms correctly (Fig. 11.2)
- communicating with trial coordinators
- reporting adverse events
- arranging safe storage of data for the statutory period
- presenting data at meetings and in peer-reviewed journals.

Research podiatrists should learn excellent presenting skills so that they can, at conferences, speak to other healthcare professionals as equals. Research gives podiatrists opportunities to promote themselves and their profession.

The downside of the role of research podiatrist is that conducting research can be tiring and time consuming and is often boring. The atmosphere of the modern National Health Service is hostile to

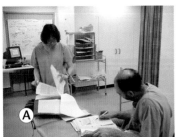
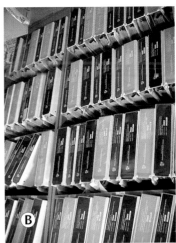

Fig. 11.2 (A) Two research podiatrists dealing with the day's paperwork generated by a research study. (B) Case record folders relating to clinical trials are space occupying and time consuming to fill in.

research. Projects are scrutinized by local and regional ethical committees and research and development committees, demanding numerous copies of projects. The amount of work taken to get a proposal accepted is often daunting and the amount of paperwork and bureaucracy involved in conducting research is sometimes overwhelming.

Funders of research into the diabetic foot include charities and pharmaceutical companies. Two great supporters of diabetic foot projects are the International Working Group on the Diabetic Foot, and the Novo Nordisk-funded World Diabetes Foundation (WDF), which was formed to develop good diabetes care in developing countries. The European Union funds research into the diabetic foot.

The WDF is currently funding a 'step by step' programme to teach basic foot care and educational skills to teams of healthcare professionals in India, Nepal, Sri Lanka, and Tanzania which, if successful, will be rolled out to other developing countries.

WORKING ABROAD

Many British podiatrists have spent time abroad to help with the management of patients with diabetes or leprosy. British podiatrists regularly visit India to help in the work of Calcutta Rescue's patients with Hansen's disease (leprosy). Gaining experience in the management of the neuropathic diabetic foot in the UK before going abroad is advisable. The late Jacquie Lloyd Roberts set up groups of very effective diabetic foot clinics in Ukraine, and her work is carried on by past and present students and staff of the Northampton School of Podiatry.

Many countries have no tradition of podiatry and British podiatrists are sometimes invited to go out and report on how a footcare service can be set up and local problems overcome. Where no local podiatrists are available, nurses and physicians can be trained in basic foot care techniques.

EXPERT WITNESSES

Podiatrists should beware of taking on the role of expert witness (see Chapter 10) unless they have extensive experience and specialist knowledge of the diabetic foot, have a broad grasp of the aetiopathology and modern developments in diagnosis and treatment, can cope with the pressures of appearing in court, can stand up to rigorous questioning, and are aware of the law relating to medical matters. They should understand the legal process and the ways in which courts work. Courses are available for podiatrists who are interested in entering this field, and the Society of Chiropodists and Podiatrists holds a list of suitable practitioners in the field who are available as experts.

FURTHER TRAINING

Further training for podiatrists in the fields of diabetes and diabetic foot care can be gained from attending courses, including the Society of Chiropodists and Podiatrists' diabetic foot module. In addition, many podiatrists are now studying for master's degrees and doctorates in diabetes or the diabetic foot.

Appendix
Useful addresses

The Society of Chiropodists and Podiatrists
1 Fellmongers' Path, Tower Bridge Road, London SE1 3LY
E-mail: enq@scpod.org

Diabetes UK
10 Parkway, London NW1 7AA
E-mail: info@diabetes.org.uk

The King's Casting Course
The Diabetic Foot Clinic, King's College Hospital NHS Trust,
Denmark Hill, Camberwell, London SE5 9RS
Tel: 0207 346 3223
E-mail: maureen.bates@kingsch.nhs.uk

The Blackburn Casting Course
Blackburn Royal Infirmary, Bolton Road, Blackburn BB2 3LR
Tel: 01254 294560

PDUK (Podiatry in Diabetes UK)
E-mail: pduk2004@hotmail.com
Web address: www.pduk.org

The International Working Group on the Diabetic Foot (IWGDF)
PO Box 9533, 1006 GA, Amsterdam, the Netherlands
E-mail: diabetic-foot@mail.com

United Kingdom Representative of IWGDF
E-mail: avmfoster@hotmail.com

Index

Note: page numbers in **bold** refer to figures or tables

E

F